Write effectively

A QUICK COURSE FOR BUSY HEALTH WORKERS

Write effectively

A QUICK COURSE FOR BUSY HEALTH WORKERS

TIM ALBERT

Radcliffe Publishing
Oxford • New York

Radcliffe Publishing Ltd
18 Marcham Road
Abingdon
Oxon OX14 1AA
United Kingdom

www.radcliffe-oxford.com

Electronic catalogue and worldwide online ordering facility.

British Library Cataloguing in Publication Data

A catalogue record for this book is available from the British Library.

ISBN-13: 978 1 84619 135 0

Typeset by Pindar New Zealand (Egan Reid), Auckland, New Zealand
Printed and bound by TJI Digital, Padstow, Cornwall, UK

Contents

About the author

Tim Albert trained as a journalist and worked on local, national and specialist health publications. In 1990 he retrained as a trainer and for the next 16 years ran more than 1000 courses on writing and editing skills for health professionals. He is a fellow of the Chartered Institute of Personnel and Development and for 10 years was a visiting fellow in medical writing at Southampton University. He is honorary president for life of the Wimereux Cricket Club in northern France. He now cultivates his garden in Surrey, writes books and rails at the world.

Prologue

This is a book about writing in which one of the main messages is stop messing about and just get on with it. So this is a very short prologue. Welcome. And get cracking.

Tim Albert
Leatherhead, July 2008

Part 1

The quick course

How this book can help

FIRST (AND EASY) TASK: Quickly write down a list of the kinds of things you have to write (e.g. reports, letters).

Many people are surprised by the range of what they have to write: reports, letters, applications, minutes, essays, protocols, policy statements, articles . . . the list goes on. They also have to face a constant procession of emails, which people tend not to count as 'real writing', but which are every bit as important – and which even the decisive can take two or more hours a day to deal with.

At the same time, many people seem particularly ill-prepared for all this writing. The task is badly defined, time-consuming and difficult. Courses on how to do it are rare. Agreement on 'good writing' seems to be rarer still, and the whole process often appears to be more about internal power squabbles than external communication. Not surprisingly, many writers in the health services dislike writing and avoid it whenever possible. Others proceed reluctantly, without confidence – and without satisfaction.

This book sets out to help you by showing you what writing is all about. It will give you some tools that will enable you to do it with more confidence. I would be lying if I said that you will come to enjoy writing (some suffering is inevitable, even desirable), but as you go through this book you should be able to approach each writing task in a more confident manner, and therefore your output should be more effective. More importantly, you should be able to take control of your writing, and once you have grasped the essentials you will have a powerful tool to help you achieve your goals.

To explain why I think this is worthwhile, I need to go into personal history. I trained and worked as a general and medical journalist, then reinvented myself nearly 20 years ago as a trainer specialising in writing and editing skills for health workers. My first course was on effective writing, and I have since run it some 300 times. Over that time it evolved markedly.

Originally, I intended to concentrate on showing participants the techniques of 'plain English', but I soon realised that this was not enough. Once I had shown them how to write simply, their bosses just changed it all back again. It was not long before I realised that their main problem was not writing *simply*, but writing *anything at all*.

Thus the main part of this book – the short course that comprises Part 1 – looks at the *process* of writing in 10 easy sessions. The aim of the first session is to start you reflecting about writing generally, and the next will give you a chance to focus on what your real writing problems are. Session 3 proposes a simple model for measuring whether writing is effective. You should then choose a piece of writing that you have to do (of any length or any subject, but the harder the better), and in the following three sessions you will be shown how to prepare for writing using three distinct planning techniques. In Session 7 you will have the chance to do some writing, and in Session 8 you will learn how to identify when the big things have gone wrong – and what you need to do to sort them out. Session 9 will identify the various micro-editing tasks you need to do on your own work, and in Session 10 you will learn how to harness the comments of other people to improve your writing.

You may wish to work through Part 1 of the book on your own, or organise a group to do it together. There are 33 tasks for you to do. Some will take just a few moments, but others will take longer. You will be developing your own work, so that by the end of the workbook you should not only know how to write effectively, you should have actually done it as well.

My intention is to provide an informal short course rather than a prolonged period of study. You will find brief bits of advice, interspersed with anecdotes and arguments that have enriched the course over the years. Where participants have tended to stop and question, I have inserted discussion points. I have also provided some tables and diagrams that I hope will be useful. I have not included long lists of references or further reading; the purpose is to get you through the 10 sessions as fast as possible – to get you *writing* rather than reading.

There are three more parts to the book. Part 2 is styled as an after-sales programme, and the intention is that you will look into it several weeks after you have finished the basic 10 steps. This part asks what problems remain (or have emerged), and gives some suggestions for future action. Part 3 deals with an important, but often neglected, part of writing: the contribution of design decisions to the effectiveness of the text.

Part 4 deals in more detail with issues of grammar and style. These are always difficult to write about, primarily because they soon become tedious and turgid for most people. My response has been to provide a series of lists on topics including parts of speech, wasteful words, fashionable clichés and useful quotes. There are also a few exercises for you to do yourself.

If you need encouragement at this stage, let me say that the ideas in this workbook have been tested over many courses, and many people have found them helpful in demystifying the writing process. I am grateful to the participant who called it 'an innovative, refreshing approach'. I definitely agree with another who wrote, 'Writing effectively involves a series of steps . . . These can be taught and learnt like any other skills' and another who stated, 'Knowing the principles of writing takes the fear out of writing.' And for one person, at least, it worked in the way I would have hoped: 'It has changed the way I write, the way I plan presentations, and my self-confidence about the messages I am trying to convey.'

And finally there was this one: 'Writing is really fun once you realise it is a big marketing game.' This should be of comfort as you go through the next nine sessions.

AT THE END OF THE WORKBOOK YOU WILL HAVE

- a thorough understanding of the areas you need to work on to make your writing more effective
- clear guidelines for measuring the success of what you have written
- easy-to-follow principles for meeting the needs of different audiences
- simple planning techniques that will reduce writer's block
- an enjoyable writing technique that will save time, reduce boredom and increase creativity
- a logical way of approaching the rewriting process, including some objective tests you can use on your draft
- a sensible strategy for making the best use of comments from colleagues and bosses.

In other words, you WILL BE ABLE TO WRITE EFFECTIVELY.

SESSION 2

So what's your real problem?

Over the years, many unhappy writers have turned up on my courses. Some have been sent because of someone else's verdict that 'they can't write'. Others still smart from humiliation inflicted by one party or another, such as teachers who told them they don't know their grammar or colleagues who said they don't know their facts, and now hate anything to do with writing. Still others are innocents: faced with a huge writing task – a scientific paper, perhaps, or a major report – they have no idea how to start. A few claim to have no writing problems, but I worry that they are deluding themselves, or lying.

The first thing to do is look more closely at why writers in the health professions seem to have so many problems. How many of their apparent shortcomings are real, and how many imagined? What are the habits that individual writers need to change, and what are requirements of the health service writing culture that they will have to learn to live with? What do they *not* need to worry about?

Your next task, therefore, is to get a better understanding of what your *real* writing problems are.

TASK 2: Go through the following statements and tick those that apply to you.
- ☐ I do not have enough time to write
- ☐ I have too many ideas
- ☐ I find it difficult to write for different types of audiences
- ☐ I find it difficult to stop researching

☐ I tend to write too much or too little
☐ I often get stuck during a writing project
☐ I spend too much time rewriting
☐ My writing tends to come back from other people full of corrections
☐ I do not know what is meant by 'good writing'
☐ I would like to be able to write more easily

WHAT IT ALL MEANS

Statement 1: I do not have enough time to write

This is by far the most common problem. Some people feel that they are failing to complete work that they should complete. (This is particularly common among those who need their work to appear in academic publications in order to advance their careers.) Others are left with the nagging feeling that, even though they have finished the writing they had to do, they would have done better if only they had a little more time. (There is rarely any objective evidence for this.) Some feel that they have to add writing to their existing duties, which means that they take work home. (They feel that this is a sign of failure as well as an intrusion.)

Solution: This is clearly a time-management issue. Writing is not an add-on, but a substantial task. It needs careful allocation of time and resources, good planning and regular application. If these are taken care of, the task becomes much easier. Time-management techniques are dealt with throughout the workbook, but particularly in Session 4.

Statement 2: I have too many ideas

Some people are bubbling with ideas. But when these ideas start to take them off in one direction, another set of ideas rears up and threatens to take them off in a different direction entirely. When they finally realise that they must stop thinking and start writing, they have no idea where to start.

Solution: Identify a specific time when you must stop thinking and start writing. This is a key phase of the planning process, and in Session 4 I outline a straightforward technique for getting started.

Statement 3: I find it difficult to write for different types of audiences

Health professionals rarely have trouble writing for their peers; that is what they have been trained to do. But they find it difficult to write for other audiences, and get positively panicky if they have to write for several audiences at the same time.

Solution: The ability to write for different types of audiences is an integral part of effective writing. In Session 3 I propose a reader-centred model that suggests you place your audience's needs at the centre of your writing, and Session 4 shows how to apply this as you start to write.

Statement 4: I find it difficult to stop researching

Some people are at their happiest when searching for information. They hope that if they persevere with their searches, Truth will emerge, and they will be ready to start writing that perfect piece (for perfect peace?). This is unlikely. This kind of behaviour is often a displacement activity (*see* the comments about writer's block, in Statement 6 below), because as long as you are researching you can delay that awful moment when you have to write.

Solution: This workbook proposes three distinct planning techniques, which are in Sessions 4, 5, and 6. These techniques should ease you gently into the writing process, while ensuring that you don't clutter your mind with too many details.

Statement 5: I tend to write too much

Those who find it difficult to stop researching also tend to write too much when they finally get going. After all, they have just collected a pile of good material and feel it would be a shame not to put it all in. But putting things in is the easy side to writing; the hard bit is deciding what to leave out.

Solution: If you want to be more efficient, you need to put in roughly the right amount of words at the first draft. This is not particularly difficult, though it does require a little planning. Again, the techniques in Sessions 4, 5 and 6 will be useful.

Statement 6: I often get stuck during a writing project

A blanket term for this is *writer's block*. If you find it difficult to stop researching (*see* question 4 above) you are suffering from *writer's block by proxy*. If you cannot get started – but instead sit for hours in an empty room, with endless cups of coffee, looking at an empty screen – you are suffering from *early onset writer's block*. With *mid-stream writer's block*, you will set off happily enough, but sooner or later the creative juices will run out and you will grind to a halt.

Solution: The antidote for all types of writer's block is to follow a logical writing process that allows you to think out where you are going before you start the writing journey, and this is covered in Sessions 4, 5 and 6.

Statement 7: I spend too much time rewriting

Some people spend hours going through what they have just written. But since many of them admit that they do not know what good writing is, they are wasting their time. Unless you have a clear idea of why you are making changes, you are fiddling with the text, not improving it.

Solution: Having a clear understanding of what effective writing is will help, and I give an achievable definition of effective writing in Session 3. Then you need to divide the rewriting/editing process into two stages: (a) addressing important weaknesses that could, if unresolved, cause the writing to fail (*see* macro-editing, Session 8), and (b) sorting out the matters of detail that you also need to get as right as possible (*see* micro-editing, Session 9).

Statement 8: My writing tends to come back from other people full of corrections

This is a common problem in the health services, where a particularly severe writing culture seems to have taken root. Writing tasks are assigned with limited instructions and few resources. When the draft is finished, all those involved with the project (and sometimes a few outsiders as well) are encouraged to get out their red pens (or the electronic equivalent) and find as much wrong with the writing as possible. It is negative, and demotivating.

Solution: Again, knowing what makes writing effective will help you keep your perspective (*see* Session 3). Because some of these criticisms are as much about retaining power as they are about refining messages, you will need some specific *upward management skills* to help you keep control. These are dealt with in Session 10.

> **TOP TIP:** The word *correction* implies that what is wrong is now being made right. But this is often clearly untrue: in many cases it is one opinion against another, and this is shown by the fact that critics often disagree, and also alter their minds over time. I prefer the word *change*. Thus we can stop saying 'our writing has been corrected' and say instead that 'our writing has been changed'. This is more accurate – and less demoralising.

Statement 9: I do not know what is meant by 'effective writing'

There seem to be as many definitions of *effective writing* as there are people trying to do it. This makes it very difficult to achieve.

Solution: Session 3 gives a clear definition of effective writing. Throughout the book there are words and phrases that should help you to build up a language so that you can discuss writing objectively with other people (who have gone through the workbook, of course!).

Statement 10: I would like to be able to write more easily

Yes, we all want this one. But I am afraid that I cannot guarantee it; in fact, a little bit of pain may be a necessary part of the process.

Solution: This book will help you to understand where the pain comes from, and show you how and when to endure it. The pleasure you will feel when your writing is finished and successful should make it all worthwhile. Honest.

TASK 3: Write down what you think your main writing problems are.

Task 3 (*continued*)

Now you have identified your real writing problems, you should be well on the way to sorting them out. Don't feel that you are the only person who suffers from them. (If you are going through this workbook with other people you should have realised this by now.)

TASK 4: In the light of the previous task, write down up to three things that you want to achieve by the end of this workbook. Also write down how you will measure your success.

1.

2.

3.

WHAT YOU HAVE ACHIEVED SO FAR

You now know what your real writing problems are – and what you need to work on to fix them.

What is effective writing?

The last session should have made clear that it is difficult to produce good writing if you don't know what good writing is. People have many (often strong) opinions on the subject: some say good writing must *flow* and others that it must be *of interest*; some say that it must be *concise* while others say it must *contain everything*; some just say they can't tell but *know it when they see it*. It is very subjective.

One of the difficulties is the use of the term *good writing*, which implies that there is a standard of excellence towards which we can aspire. That's fine if we know and agree what that standard is, but that rarely happens. I prefer the term *effective writing*; it implies that the writing is there to do a task, and its success (or failure) can be measured by whether it does it (or does not do it). This leads to the following uncontroversial definition:

> Effective writing gets your message across to your target audience.

This definition allows us to focus clearly on a particular type of writing, and means that various types of writing are outside our scope, such as the following:

1 *Political writing:* This type of writing is intentionally unclear: the aim is *not* to put a message across clearly. Politicians often use this technique, as do bureaucratic institutions, such as the grant-giving organisation that did not want to say *no*, so wrote saying

instead that *the application has been administratively inactivated.* (Senior health professionals can be extremely good at political writing, though for it to count as a skill it needs to have been done deliberately.)

2 *Literature:* This is not so much concerned with putting messages across as with satisfying the need of authors to write. For most people the work will lie largely unread; for the few greats such as Shakespeare and Yeats it will be read by millions. If you want to explore the art of writing literature, go to a creative writing class. This workbook is about writing as a craft, not an art: the aim is not to uncover basic truths about the human condition but to put basic messages across (to improve the human condition, one would hope, but that's another story).

1 THE READER-CENTRED MODEL FOR EFFECTIVE WRITING

If the purpose of effective writing is to put messages across, then that leads to a simple model (*see* below). In this model we have a *writer* who has a *message* and wishes to put it across to a *target audience.* For instance, John sends an email to Janet arranging to meet at the Writer's Arms public house.

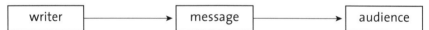

FIGURE 3.1 Effective writing model

Yet, as we all know, the process does not always run smoothly, and John is sometimes left to drink alone. The reason is that there is a 'brick wall' between the message and the audience (*see* Figure 3.2 below). Audiences have interesting and important things to do (Janet might be composing a love sonnet, or working on her PhD), and are not waiting to leap upon every piece of writing that passes by. As a writer, you must work to get your audience involved, and if you fail to do so, you have wasted your time (and possibly some trees as well).

There is a useful mnemonic here: **PIANO.**

Put
It
Across
Not
Out

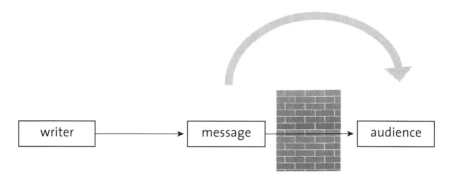

FIGURE 3.2 Effective writing model (revision 1)

How do you increase your chances of getting your message over the brick wall? There are two tricks. The first is to stop seeing everything from the perspective of the writer ('What do I want to put in?'), and start considering the needs, wants, attitudes and skills of the target audience ('What's the best way of putting this so that the audience will be interested and understand?').

The second trick is to have a clear view of your target audience. Narrow it down as far as possible: if you are writing to be published in a journal or magazine, for instance, the target audience should be the editor who makes that decision. If you are writing a proposal for a new service initiative, the target audience should be those who make that decision. If you are writing a thesis, the target audience should be the examiner.

Being clear about the target audience means that you can carry out *market research* in advance: what kind of writing have he/she/they liked in the past? What do they read? How do they write? This will provide valuable information to help you put your message across the wall.

2 THE PAY-OFF

Now we get to the crucial bit – the pay-off. This will vary from one piece of writing to another. The pay-off for John will be that Janet meets him in the right pub at the right time. With a journal article, the pay-off will be that the article is accepted; for a new service application it will be that you get the required funding; for a thesis it will be that you pass (or if you are particularly ambitious, that you pass with distinction).

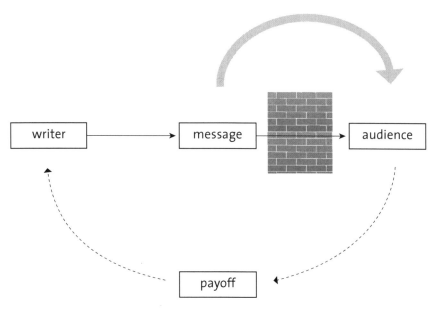

FIGURE 3.3 Effective writing model (revision 2)

Your writing will often have pleasant consequences for you, such as citations, admiration from colleagues or even that warm rosy glow that comes from thinking you may have created a masterpiece. You will also face negative consequences, such as criticisms of your grammar and spelling, complaints about the turgidity of your prose or dossiers on alleged errors. But these are distractions; the real measure is not so much what people think as whether your writing meets its objective. The fact that there is a split infinitive in paragraph 17 does not mean you are a rubbish writer, particularly if your report has brought you the £300,000 grant you wanted.

This model is extremely flexible, because it allows you to set your own goal for your writing, depending on the context. For instance, if you are dealing with a letter of complaint, your target audience will normally be the person who complains and the pay-off will be that they stop complaining. However, if the complaint is particularly explosive, you might choose instead to define the target audience as the judge in some future trial, and the pay-off will be that you (or your employer) avoid a massive payout in the courts. To take another example, if your boss is unable to explain the purpose of the writing task (as in, for example, an annual report of public health), you may decide to make your boss the target audience, with the pay-off achieved when he or she approves the work. (If you have to do this with everything you write, however, bear in mind that with a job application letter the audience is whoever is making up the shortlist, and the pay-off is getting on that list.)

DISCUSSION POINT: 'But there are often many audiences . . .'

A common objection to this model is that in the health services many documents have to serve a number of different audiences at the same time. My reaction to this objection is that it probably explains why so many health service documents fail to have any effect. By trying to meet the needs of so many diverse people and interest groups, they end up satisfying none.

There is a solution: *layering*. Instead of trying to make one document work for several audiences, produce several documents, and target each at a particular audience – with a particular pay-off in mind. Each may have to be written in a different style, and each could vary in structure (*see* Session 6). Producing a report advocating the establishment of a new clinic could give you the following layers:

- *Report:* This will be the central document. The target audience will be colleagues in your field, and the pay-off will be that they judge the report to be sound and decide to support its aims.
- *Executive summary:* The target audience will be the decision makers on the committee, and the pay-off will be that they implement your recommendation (for example, by giving you the funds you are asking for).
- *Appendix:* The target audience will be those who like plenty of data, and the pay-off will be that they find enough information to enable them to go away happy and support your report.
- *Letter:* You could write to a patient support group explaining precisely how your proposal will benefit them, and your pay-off will be that they give you their support. By all means send them the full report, but for them the report should be considered the supporting document, not the primary one.

Some people fear that layering is time-consuming. I disagree. Writing a small number of well-targeted pieces is easier than trying to make one piece fit all. And there's no greater waste of time than writing a document that no one understands.

TASK 5: Think of a document you had trouble writing recently and write the details down in the space below. Could you have layered it? Would that have made it easier and more effective?

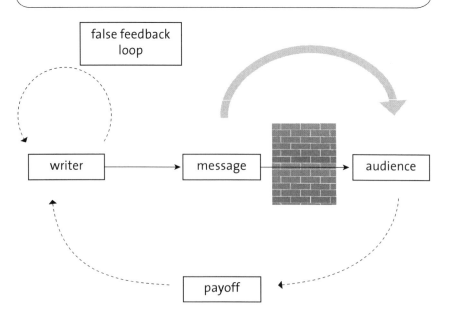

FIGURE 3.4 Effective writing model (final version)

3 FALSE FEEDBACK LOOP

Now let's add a complication – the *false feedback loop*.

It is best explained by example. A practice nurse prepares a leaflet for patients giving some useful health advice. When it is finished, the practice nurse will pass it to one of the senior GPs for comments; they will use their medical knowledge to make the document more 'medically sound'. It will then go to one of the younger GPs, who will use their more recently acquired knowledge and their commitment to 'evidence-based medicine' to make a different set of changes. Finally it will go to one of the more vociferous patients, who will make use of their commitment to patients' autonomy and dignity to make sure there is nothing that could possibly cause offence.

This is the false feedback loop. A document that has been carefully prepared for one audience is being altered by people who aren't part of that audience, with a strong risk that it ends up unfit for purpose. (This is probably another reason why so many official health service documents are unreadable: they go through so many hoops that, while they end up pleasing the committee that wrote them, the target audiences find them incomprehensible.)

These false feedback loopers are not just colleagues, partners and supervisors. One of the most dangerous sources of false feedback is you, the writer. The temptation is to write what you happen to think is good, rather than what the audience will read and understand. Resist the temptation: write for the reader, not for yourself.

This is not to say that all inputs from other people have no value and should be ignored, because that is clearly untrue. But when writing, you must be careful to accept changes that will help the message get through – and reject those that will obscure it.

4 A NEW DEFINITION OF EFFECTIVE WRITING

At the start of this chapter, I gave the following definition: effective writing gets your message across to the target audience. I now offer a new, complementary, definition.

> Effective writing is a tool that helps us to achieve what we want to achieve.

It is not about personality, or education or any other personal quality. It is, quite simply, about whether the writing works. This means being absolutely clear about what you are trying to do, and why. This will be the topic of the next session.

TASK 6: Write down a few pieces of writing you have completed recently. With the benefit of hindsight, ask what the goal of each should have been, and whether you met those goals.

WHAT YOU HAVE ACHIEVED SO FAR

You now have a clear – and measurable – concept of effective writing.

Getting started – the brief

Many people start the writing process by pulling out all the relevant information they can find and placing it in little piles around the computer (on desks, on chairs and on the floor). They then type in a title and – after a pause to gather their thoughts – start writing furiously. When they finally run out of steam, they realise that they have written too much, so they start taking out bits and pieces, rearranging whole sections, and fretting over the details.

This is like piling up a load of bricks and shaping them into a house: it may work in the end, but it is the long way. What you need is good planning, and I will recommend three separate phases. These should reduce the amount of time you have to spend on your writing. They should also increase your chances of putting your message across.

The first of these phases involves *setting the brief*. Its purpose is to define five essential elements of the writing task – in other words, a *product specification*.

> TASK 7: Identify a piece of writing you wish to work on. You should have already done the research/information gathering. Take a quick look at this information – then put it away!

Putting away the information before you start writing can be scary, like throwing away a favourite teddy bear. But there is a point to it. You will probably have gathered too much information. If you keep it all beside you, you will be constantly distracted, and tempted to put it all in. If you put it away, you will be able to focus on the main points, and your memory will help you to select the main things you need to say to support them. You will almost certainly leave something out, but it will probably be minor and you will have a chance to put it in later.

1 THE MESSAGE

The first of the five components you need to make decisions on is the message. In this context, a message is the main point that you wish to put across to the target reader. For example:

▮ *We need to close a ward.*
▮ *This patient needs a blood test.*
▮ *Eating five portions of vegetables a day will protect you against ingrowing toenails.*
▮ *Bananas can help you give up smoking.*

The message has three important characteristics:

(i) It must be single
If you want your reader to go away with one clear message, then you need to be clear in advance what that message is. The following statement has two messages: *Bananas taste delicious and are an excellent way of giving up smoking.* It is fine as far as it goes, but it could be simpler and more focused, If you want your writing to be clear, you need to be focused. Are you trying to say:

   Bananas taste delicious, or
   Bananas are an excellent tool for giving up smoking, or (if you want a message that will combine the two)
   Bananas have fantastic properties, or even
   We all need to eat more bananas?

If you can't decide, how do you expect the reader to? If you really do have two messages of equal importance, then you should think about doing two pieces of writing.

(ii) It must have a verb
Being short and single is not enough; the message must include a verb (what was called at school the 'doing word' – or what the Dutch call the *werkwoord*, literally the word that does the work).

- *Bananas* prevent *people from giving up smoking.*
- *Bananas* are not tasted *by people who give up smoking.*
- *Bananas* are not bought *by people who give up smoking.*
- *Eat bananas and your desire for smoking* will go away.

WARNING: Phrases that look like messages but aren't!

The following lack a verb and therefore are too vague to act as messages:

- *To look into the relationship between bananas and smoking.* This may be the right place to start a *project* because it sets out what you have to do. But when it comes to the actual writing you need to be further forward, and to have come to some kind of conclusion (message).
- *Do bananas help people stop smoking?* This is a question. Questions are good, but if you want to write clearly you need to have the answer before you start.
- *Bananas and smoking cessation: a multi-centre international study.* This is a *title.* It is something you add at the end of your writing to indicate to readers what you have written (or even better, why they should read it). But the custom is to write what you are looking at (and sometimes how you looked at it), but not what you found or decided (the message). Again this is not precise enough to help you at this stage.

(iii) It should be expressed in everyday language

Keep the message simple. *Bananas prevent people from giving up smoking* rather than *Regular banana consumption has an inhibitive effect on tobacco withdrawal programmes.* It does not have to appear in simple language in the final version (and sadly the conventions are that it rarely does). But at this stage you will find it helpful if you can think in the language you would use in the pub or shower. Far from being 'anti-scientific', this technique will force you to be more precise: if you are using short and precise words it is much harder to get away with vagueness.

Play around with your message. Write it down, and then challenge it yourself. If you come up with another version, write that down as well. Ask others what they think (this is particularly useful if you are writing with co-authors). You may find the message evolving and getting clearer. You may also find that you end up with the message you first thought of. Don't worry; it means you have tested it thoroughly.

When you are content with your message, you will have completed the most difficult and important part of writing – working out what you want to say. Doing this *before* writing rather than *during* or *after* will save considerable time later.

> TASK 8: Put this workbook down and do something else, such as get on a bicycle, go for a walk or take a bath. While you do this, start thinking gently about the message you want to give. When you are satisfied, write it down; aim for about 10 words – with a verb.

2 THE 'MARKET'

You now need to be clear about whom you are aiming your message at – and how you are going to reach them. Be as specific as possible. This will enable you to make wise decisions over such issues as length, tone and even individual words. Find out what your audience needs, values and reads, and this will help you with your subsequent decisions.

When you know *whom* you want to reach, the next question is *how*. There are many alternatives: an email, a letter, a report, an executive summary, a journal article, a leaflet, a newsletter, a message in a bottle and so on. Ask yourself which medium is most likely to get the message across to the target audience.

> DISCUSSION POINT: A solution for the jargon problem
> Some of what is called *jargon* is simply sloppy, overblown writing: *the lower limbs of the male paediatric patients* rather than *the boys' legs*. But most of the time it is what the writer has come to accept as normal technical language but which is unfamiliar to the target audience. The phrases *myocardial infarct* and *competency framework* are fine when writing for fellow professionals (members of the same tribe), for whom they will have a proper technical meaning. But as soon as you start writing for other audiences, they will not understand. So jargon

is basically *technical language used inappropriately.* If you follow the technique in this workbook, the problem should go away, because one of the first things you are encouraged to do is define clearly your target audience. If you do your job properly you will choose the right language for them. Simple.

TASK 9: Write down your market (target audience), and how you will reach them.

---

3 THE LENGTH/FORMAT

How long should a piece of writing be? People sometimes assume that the length should reflect the 'importance' of the topic. This is a fallacy, because it is based on the writer's needs, not those of the audience. In reality, the length often just reflects how much information the author has collected on the topic. The correct answer is (in theory at least) simple: whatever length your target audience will be comfortable with.

TASK 10: Write down the approximate number of words your piece of writing should have.

4 THE DEADLINE

When will you finish your piece of writing? Deciding on a deadline (and putting it in your diary) right at the beginning is one of the best things you can do to ensure that your writing gets finished. Allow yourself a reasonable amount of time, and, if your writing depends on the cooperation of others, build in a little slack.

For major projects, one deadline is not enough; you need to write a schedule – a succession of mini-deadlines.

Set brief	January 14
Complete first draft	January 18
Send polished draft to others	January 24
Polished draft back from others	January 27
PUBLISH*	January 29

*I use this term to mean when the piece of writing is completed and sent out to be read by the audience, for example when a letter is posted, a report is placed in the internal mail or the SEND button is pressed.

FIGURE 4.1 Example of a schedule

If others are involved, you should try to get them to agree in advance to your schedule. But make sure you meet the dates yourself; if you are late, they will not hesitate to follow your example.

TASK 11: Fill in the schedule for the project you are working on.

Set brief

Complete first draft

Send polished draft to others

Polished draft back from others

PUBLISH

5 THE PAY-OFF

I have defined effective writing as a tool for achieving a specific goal. So before you start writing you must be sure you know what your goal is – and how you can measure whether it has been met. This becomes the *pay-off*. Has the money been granted? Have the recommendations been accepted? Has the complainant gone away? If you achieve your goal, your writing has been effective.

Make sure that the combination of message and market is able to deliver the required pay-off. The following will probably fail:

Message: the health authority should fund a banana therapy clinic
Market: public via a leaflet
Pay-off: we get funds to set up the clinic

Whether public opinion is in favour of the clinic is not really the point; you need the funding and that is not theirs to give. The following two alternatives, however, would have a chance of succeeding:

Message: the health authority should fund a banana therapy clinic
Market: public via a leaflet
Pay-off: public opinion is in favour

Message: the health authority should fund a banana therapy clinic
Market: health authority executive
Pay-off: funds to set up the clinic

By the time you have thought through all five elements of the brief, you should have a clear idea of how you will solve this particular writing task. And the clearer – and more focused – you are at this stage, the easier the rest of the writing task will be. The hard work is already done. With reasonable luck you will find that you have turned what could have been a long and arduous voyage of discovery into a brief pleasure trip.

TASK 12: Set the brief.
Now bring together the five elements to create a brief for your writing ...

Message

Market

Length

Deadline

Pay-off

TOP TIP: Getting agreement

The decisions you have made at this early stage will help you keep focused on completing the task, and they should also help you to reduce the amount of refocusing (and fiddling about) in the later stages.

Make sure that others who have an interest in your writing (your boss, your boss's boss, your colleagues, your contributors) know about your brief. Send them a copy, and try to get them to agree at this stage; if they cannot agree now they are unlikely to do so later.

TASK 13: Show your brief to a co-author or supervisor. Record their reactions.

WHAT YOU HAVE ACHIEVED SO FAR

You have now defined what you are writing, for whom, when and why. All you now have to do is add several hundred (or thousand) words. The most important bit is over.

SESSION 5

Sorting the information

You have now decided what you are going to write, for whom, when and why. One way forward would be to start jotting down a list of all the things you want to say. This works up to a point, but there is always the danger that you will start to lose focus. Lists have a tendency to charge off in a particular direction, from where you may find it difficult to change or return. They can also make it difficult for you to see potential relationships, since in a list each item is related only to the one before and the one after. At this stage it pays to have a little more flexibility.

I strongly recommend doing a *spidergram*. This technique can be done quickly and allows you to keep focusing clearly on the message, yet at the same time is flexible. You need to set aside about 10 minutes. (I recommend using a kitchen timer as an aid to concentration). Take a large piece of paper, set out lengthways; put your message in the centre; and then draw a line around it, as in the following.

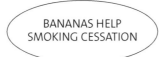

FIGURE 5.1 Spidergram step 1

> TASK 14: Take a blank piece of paper and start a spidergram by writing your message in the middle.

Now you must establish four or five main points or questions that you need to ask in order to flesh out this message. Often you can use some or all of Kipling's 'honest serving men': *who? what? where? when? why?* and *how?* plus (an extra one) *so what?* You may find specific questions more suitable: *Why do we need smoking cessation? Why is giving up smoking so hard? How can bananas help? What should we do about it?*

> TASK 15: Write a small number of questions around the central message, and connect each of them to the centre with a line (*see* below).

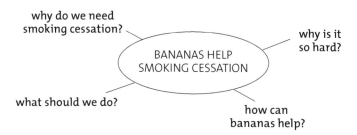

FIGURE 5.2 Spidergram step 2

When you have done this, take one of the questions and start writing down what comes into your mind, making sure that you use single ideas, not phrases or sentences: *bruised yellow banana* should be *banana* with two qualifiers *bruised* and *yellow*. When you later realise it was also *half eaten* you can add that as well; and you can qualify the bruising with, say, the colour of the bruising, how it was done, etc.

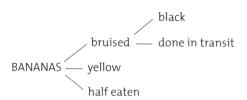

FIGURE 5.3 Building the spidergram

The ideas should be branching out one by one like this.

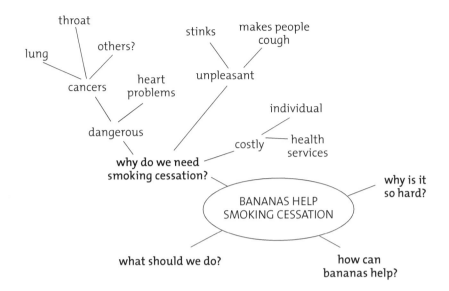

FIGURE 5.4 Spidergram step 3

They should not be lumped together like this.

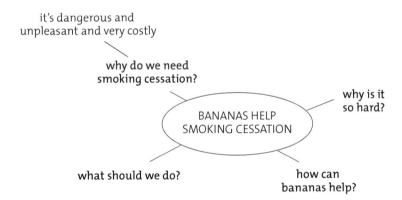

FIGURE 5.5 Spidergram gone wrong

When you have exhausted one line of thought, go back to the beginning and start again. Work out from the middle. Make sure that there is a line going back to the middle. Do not have ideas 'floating' (if they are floating they can't be relevant to the message, however attached you might be to them). Do not be too critical: at this stage you should be capturing ideas rather than evaluating them.

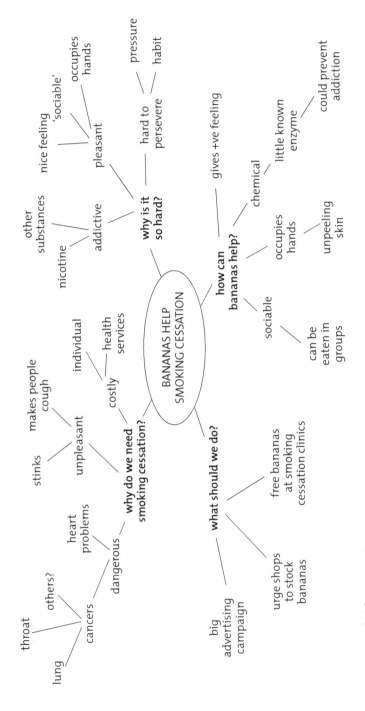

FIGURE 5.6 Spidergram step 4

TOP TIP: Use the sections of your writing as a basis for your questions

If you are writing a major piece of work, you can formulate your main questions to coincide with the main sections you envisage. For instance, with scientific papers there are four sections, which ask the following questions:

- Why did we start?
- What did we do?
- What did we find?
- What does it mean?

This gives an excellent framework for a spidergram. A similar approach can be used, for example, with a major report or even with a book.

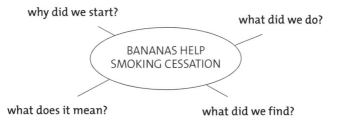

FIGURE 5.7 New spidergram step 1

So what have you achieved after 10 minutes? First, you will have plenty of ideas written down on your piece of paper. Since they can all be traced back to the middle, they are all directly related not to the subject as a whole, but to the particular message you want to put across. What you have left out is as important as what you have put in. Second, these ideas are now out in the open. As a course participant once remarked, 'The mess in my head is now the mess on a piece of paper.' That's progress.

A useful analogy is that of building a tree. One wouldn't build a tree by shuffling leaves around, yet this is in effect how many people write. They collect the facts, shuffle them about, and hope that a good shape emerges. The sensible option would be to start with the tree trunk, then the branches. After this it becomes straightforward to hang out the leaves. This is what we have done: build up from the centre.

Some people find this difficult, and certainly it's not compulsory. But others find it a revelation, because it helps them to organise their information and clarify their thinking. At the same time it shows up

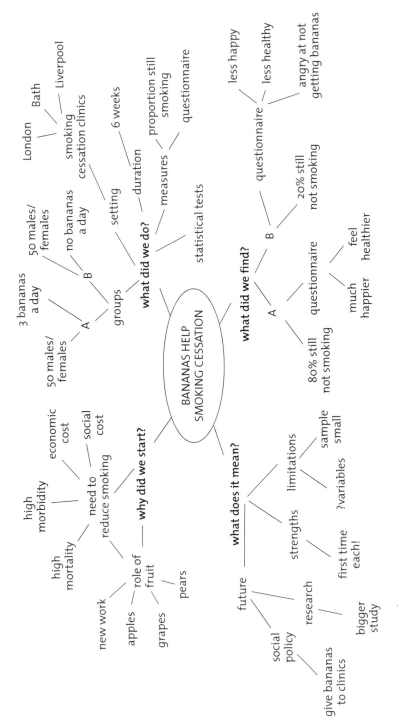

FIGURE 5.8 New spidergram step 2

gaps of knowledge that need to be filled. It is an *information processing* activity, a prelude to a linear list rather than a substitute for one. Writing this list – or drawing up the plan – will be dealt with in the next session.

WHAT YOU HAVE ACHIEVED SO FAR

You have now sorted information that could be used in your writing.

Putting together a plan

Writing has content and structure. By now you should be familiar with the information you could use as content; the next step is to work out which bits of information, and in which order, you actually will use. This normally involves making a plan, but to do it well (and relatively easily) it helps to understand two things:

▌ how sentences are grouped together in paragraphs, which are the basic building blocks of writing and have a particular structure

▌ how these building blocks fit together to make an overall structure for a piece of writing.

1 PARAGRAPH STRUCTURE

Writing is made up of words, grouped together into sentences, grouped together into paragraphs. Each paragraph has about five sentences, and can be considered the basic building block of writing. Each paragraph should advance the piece of writing. When it comes to writing a paragraph, there is an important principle: the first sentence is crucial, and should give the direction (or message) of that paragraph. The remaining sentences elaborate, explain and add evidence. School children in the United States have formal lessons on writing these important first sentences, which they call *topic sentences*. For instance:

▌ *It's a lovely day today. The sky is blue. The sun is shining. The birds are singing, etc.*

▌ *But tomorrow it will be worse. The rain is coming in from the east, etc.*

■ ***But then it will clear for the weekend.*** *As another piece of high pressure comes in from Ireland. And the birds will be back singing in the trees, etc.*

This can be represented visually as an *inverted triangle* (*see* below), in which the main point comes first, and then the supporting information comes in decreasing order of importance.

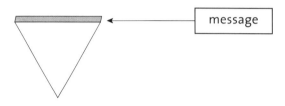

FIGURE 6.1 Well-structured paragraph

Provided that the topic sentence in the first paragraph logically leads on to the topic sentence in the second paragraph, and the topic sentence in the second paragraph logically leads on to the topic sentence in the third paragraph (and so on), your writing will flow.

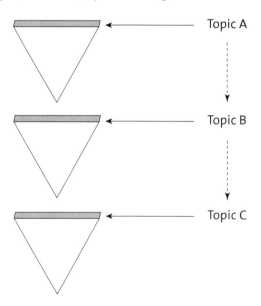

FIGURE 6.2 Well-structured and flowing paragraphs

Some people feel (or have been taught) that writing will flow only if they manage to link the last sentence of each paragraph with the first of the next. This is extremely difficult to do; it is also unnecessary, particularly since many people will be scanning the piece of writing rather than going through sentence by sentence.

2 OVERALL STRUCTURE

When it comes to considering whole pieces of writing, the same question recurs: where do you put the message? One commonly used structure keeps to the inverted triangle principle. Another does the opposite, and puts the message at the end. A third uses a combination of the two. There are, of course, other ways to structure a piece of writing, but these three will do for most occasions.

(i) The inverted triangle
This structure is based on the reasonable assumption that the one sentence people are most likely to read is the first one, so you should put your message there. Once you have done that, add the rest of your information in decreasing order of importance.

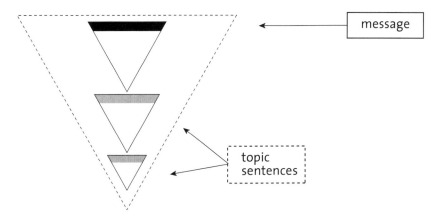

FIGURE 6.3 Overall structure: inverted triangle

Some people (particularly those trained in the sciences) feel that this is a sensational approach. But I am talking about *where the message goes*, and not *what the message says*. It goes without saying that the message should be accurate, reasonable and supported by the evidence. In fact, the structure discourages sensationalism, because it forces writers to be absolutely clear (and literally upfront) about their message, rather than making it vague or burying it so that no one notices.

This structure is appropriate for the following types of writing: emails, letters, executive summaries, news stories, press releases and other short communications.

(ii) The scientific paper (IMRAD)

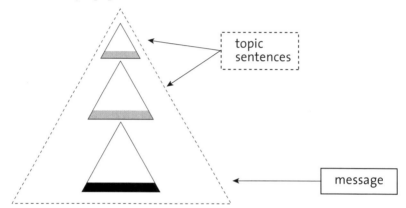

FIGURE 6.4 Overall structure: IMRAD

This is the kind of structure with which scientists tend to be most comfortable. It is based on the *IMRAD* structure of scientific papers: Introduction, Method, Results and Discussion. It generally starts with an introduction to the topic (*Smoking cessation is generally considered to be a priority for public health*). It then goes on to describe the method used to investigate the topic, followed by the data generated. Finally it goes on to discuss the meaning and relevance of it all, ending with the implication of the study, in other words the message (*Bananas give us a new way of helping smokers to stop*).

In this model, the message should appear at the end (though, alas, it does not always). Leaving the message until last is taking a big risk: what are the chances of the reader actually getting that far? In communication terms, this structure is not particularly effective, but it is appropriate whenever the audience expects it.

This structure is appropriate for the following types of writing: scientific articles, some reports and some academic work.

DISCUSSION POINT: Where should the message go?

Medicine information pharmacists face an interesting dilemma over how to structure their letters. Part of their work involves replying to queries from GPs, such as *If I give product x and product y to my patient, will they die?* Their scientific training leads many of them to structure their letter in the IMRAD style.

■ Paragraph one: *Thank you for your interesting inquiry about drugs x and y ...*
■ Paragraph two: *I have looked at a number of databases to find the answer ...*
■ Paragraph three: *I found a number of important studies ...*
■ Paragraph four: *Prescribing product x and product y together will kill your patient.*

In other words, the message comes at the end (IMRAD). An alternative is to put the message at the beginning (inverted triangle):

■ Paragraph one: *Prescribing product x and product y together will kill your patient.*
■ Paragraph two: *I found a number of important studies ...*
■ Paragraph three: *I have looked at a number of databases to find the answer ...*
■ Paragraph four: *Thank you for your interesting inquiry blah blah blah ...*

This brought hours of argument in my courses, as many pharmacists insisted that the latter structure is far too vulgar. Once when there was a group of GPs on the same course, I asked them which structure they would prefer. Unanimously they voted for the second: 'We want the answer quickly,' they said, 'and don't want to spend time ploughing through the waffle.'

(iii) The hourglass

One limitation of the inverted triangle structure is that if the article is longer than a few hundred words it needs something a little more sophisticated to keep the reader interested. This leads us to what has been called the 'hourglass' structure, which is a combination of the inverted triangle and IMRAD.

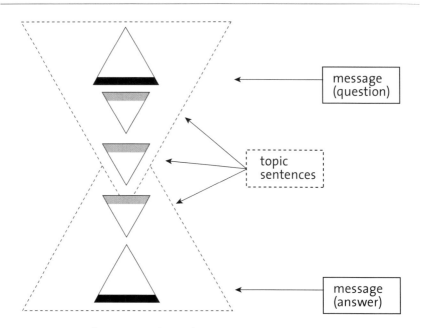

FIGURE 6.5 Overall structure: hourglass

This structure has three components. In the introduction, the purpose is to attract the reader's interest – and to set up a *dynamic* (or question) that will help to ensure that this interest is maintained throughout (*So how can bananas help us give up smoking?*). After this comes the *development*, in which the writing proceeds, paragraph by paragraph, to answer this question. Finally comes the *conclusion*, which is the answer to the question – and the message (*Bananas really can help us give up smoking*). In other words, the message comes in twice: in question form at the start of the piece of writing, and as a statement at the end.

This structure is appropriate for the following types of writing: newspaper feature articles, some reports, book chapters and journal editorials.

TASK 16: Use the information in the following press release to write a news article for the *Wormwood Newsletter*. This publication is read by all staff members, from kitchen staff to directors.

Wormwood University Hospital has appointed the new Financial Controller. Mr John Smith commenced on 17 January and his main responsibilities will be:

- financial advice to the Director of Finance
- control of the hospital's internal administrative budget
- all payments to contractors
- financial control of all budgets
- internal audit.

Mr Smith qualified in 1995 as a Chartered Accountant whilst working for Arthur Andersen & Co. after which he spent approximately nine years with Associated Chemicals Plc in a variety of Financial Controller roles.

After spending a year as the Finance Director with a Computer Reservation Company he is pleased to be joining the medical world.

He lives with his wife and two daughters in Silchester, England. A keen sportsman, he has represented Great Britain at judo many times, and was European champion for three years.

Task 16 (*continued*)

There are a number of ways of starting this piece of writing. The most common first sentence is the straightforward: *John Smith has been appointed the new financial controller*. This is accurate, but dull. Then there is: *We are pleased to announce the appointment of John Smith as financial controller.* This is not only dull (and writer-centred rather than reader-centred) but also smacks of propaganda. (They would be pleased – they made the appointment).

Some people go to the end of the press release for their opening: *A judo champion has been appointed financial controller* or, to take it further still, *It's going to be difficult to floor our new financial controller – he's a judo champion!* This can attract charges of sensationalism. But it is not saying anything that isn't in the press release; it is simply taking what the target audience is likely to find interesting (or least boring) and putting it at the top of the article. If the object is to get people interested, then it must be a sensible decision.

3 WRITING THE PLAN

Understanding how pieces of writing can be structured will help enormously when it comes to writing the plan. There are three stages.

(i) Decide on the length
Take a view on how long the piece of writing should be, or, to be more specific, what your target audience will bear. Word counts are rather vague. You will probably find it more useful to think about numbers of paragraphs. (A letter will commonly have three or four; a scientific paper typically has four sections with 2-7-7-6 paragraphs per section.)

(ii) Work out what goes into each paragraph
Decide the overall structure (i.e. where your message will go). Then decide what each paragraph will deal with. It is worth referring back to the spidergram for inspiration.

(iii) Write down your plan on a piece of paper
Make a brief note of what each paragraph will deal with. This is definitely not the same as writing down what each paragraph will contain. At this stage, it is important to keep it general – so that we can unleash some creative powers (yes, really) in the next step.

Plan	Plan
Discussion	1. Intro: bananas could be a breakthrough in smoking cessation
1. What we found	2. Why smoking cessation has been a problem
2. Limitations	3. How bananas can help
3. Strengths	4. What should we do about it
4. Context	
5. Implications for research	
6. Implications for practice	

FIGURE 6.6 Two short plans

TASK 17: Write a short plan for the piece of work you are working on.

WHAT YOU HAVE ACHIEVED SO FAR

▌ You know how to write a simple and effective paragraph.
▌ You know how to choose an appropriate overall structure.
▌ You know how to draft a short and effective plan.

Writing the first draft – and enjoying it!

Now is the time to start writing. All you need are three things:

▌ the plan
▌ an implement (computer, pen, pencil or dictating machine)
▌ peace and quiet.

Your plan is done. An implement should be easy to find. As for peace and quiet . . . that might be a little harder. In today's working environment, few people have offices to themselves, so finding a quiet corner for, say, a couple of interruption-free hours is usually out of the question.

If you can't write in a busy office, you need a strategy, such as coming in early, writing at home (though here it can be harder to resist distractions) or slipping off to an empty meeting room (or the loo). Some of these may only be viable for short periods of time, such as 10–15 minutes. The good – but no doubt surprising – news is that this is all the time you need.

1 FREE WRITING

With the technique of *free writing*, you sit down with just your plan beside you, and let rip. You start with the first sentence, and as soon as you have written that you continue with the second. Under no circumstances should you look back and start playing about with what you have already written. If there are details you don't know, leave a gap and fill them in later. If there are references, again make a note and put them in later. The key at this stage is, to adapt a quote attributed to the American humorist James Thurber, not to get it right, but to get it written. If you keep your discipline, you should be able to do 300 words in 10 minutes, as countless course participants have found, somewhat to their surprise. This is enough for a one-page executive summary or the introduction to a scientific paper.

Why do it this way? First, when we write we need to be both *critical* and *creative*. You have already gone through three planning procedures (the brief, the spidergram and the plan) where you had many opportunities to be critical. Now is the time to be creative. Let your writing flow, and you may well be surprised by how far you get. Second, writing in one short burst will enable you to keep the shape and flow of what you are writing far more effectively than if you keep going away and coming back. And finally, you might enjoy yourself – many people have reported that they do when free writing. Apart from being desirable in its own right, this enjoyment will rub off on the readers.

Once your time runs out, don't start reading what you have written. Put it down, walk away and do not to come back to it until at least the following day.

> TASK 18: Clear your desk, make sure your original material is put away, and start writing. Continue for 10 minutes. Then stop.

Many people feel that anything they have done so quickly is unlikely to be of value. Actually, it wasn't that quick if you consider the planning that preceded it. Nevertheless, you now need to test your hypothesis that this draft is of little value, and we will do this is the next session. You could be pleasantly surprised.

WHAT YOU HAVE ACHIEVED SO FAR

You can now be creative – and fast – when you write the first draft.

Rewriting – asking the Big Five Questions

Out of many thousands of people who came on my courses, only one has refused point-blank to entertain the idea of rewriting. Most people realise that it an integral part of the process, so it is a pity it is often done so badly. We tend to fiddle with the more obvious bits (particularly style), but fail to ask the really important questions. In order to ensure that these are given the priority they deserve, I have divided the rewriting process into two stages: *macro-editing* and *micro-editing*.

Macro-editing, which is the subject of this session, requires the author to consider five key questions:

▎ Does your writing contain a clear *message*?
▎ Do you still want to put that message across to the target audience (*market*)?
▎ Is that message supported by the *evidence*?
▎ Is the *structure* appropriate for that audience?
▎ Is the *tone* appropriate for that audience?

When you start revising, the first thing to do is read your draft, and then apply these questions. They will not be difficult to answer (though you may not always get the answer you are hoping for). There are some tests that you can use, and once you have answered the five questions satisfactorily, you can be confident that your writing is almost ready to send on its way. (Some polishing will be needed, but that will be dealt with in Session 9).

QUESTION 1: IS THERE A MESSAGE?

Writing commonly fails because the reader has no idea what the author is trying to say. So the first Big Question is whether the message you identified at the brief-setting stage is still in there somewhere. Look for *where* your message actually appears. If it is at the beginning or the end of the piece (depending on your readers' preferred habits), you will have done well. If it appears elsewhere, you should consider whether to move it to the top or bottom, and if it is hard to find the message, you will need to consider rewording it to make it more explicit. None of this should be difficult.

QUESTION 2: DO YOU STILL WANT TO PUT THAT MESSAGE ACROSS TO THE TARGET AUDIENCE (MARKET)?

Unless circumstances have suddenly changed (or you have taken an unreasonably long time to get this far), your answer should be yes. This is not surprising, because you thought carefully about message and market *before* you started writing. This early work is now paying dividends.

If your answer is no to this question (though if you do the preparation well such incidents should be very few and far between), you will have to go back and work on a revised brief. You may also need to have a word with the person who gave you the task of writing the piece in the first place.

QUESTION 3: IS YOUR MESSAGE SUPPORTED BY THE EVIDENCE?

At this stage we are not concerned with methodological minutiae, or even with accuracy. But you do need to satisfy yourself that your message is adequately supported. The arguments should be clear and logical, and there should be no obvious loopholes. If you feel that your case is reasonable, move on to the next question. If you feel there are problems, make a note of them and make sure they are dealt with at the micro-editing stage.

QUESTION 4: IS YOUR STRUCTURE APPROPRIATE?

One simple but useful test is to count the paragraphs and make sure that they are within the bounds of what the target audience will bear.

A second test is to look at the paragraph structure. How does it flow? Is it confusing? Is it likely to take the reader along to the end? Take a yellow marker pen and go through what you have written. Highlight the 'important' sentences, so that someone who read only these would get a good idea of what you are trying to say. Identify whole sentences only. When you have done it, look at where the yellow sentences are appearing.

(i) At the beginning: If you are consistently highlighting the first sentence of each paragraph, you can relax. It means that you are following the inverted triangle structure explained in Session 6 and starting each paragraph with the topic sentence. This is good news.

(ii) At the end: If the highlighted (i.e. important) sentences are coming in at the end of a paragraph, the piece of writing is likely to be difficult to read. This is not good news: consider revamping your paragraphs so that these key sentences appear at the beginning.

(iii) In the middle: If the highlighted sentences are coming in the middle of a paragraph, you also need to consider remedial action. It seems as if these sentences are being needlessly buried. Consider moving them to the top of each paragraph. Alternatively, consider this sentence the starting point of each new paragraph, with the preceding sentences moving up into the previous paragraph.

(iv) Absent: If there is a paragraph with no highlighted sentence, why is that paragraph there? If you can think of no good reason, strike it out. If you feel it is important, write a topic sentence that will explain why it is important.

(v) Omnipresent: If you have highlighted several sentences in a paragraph, then you need to consider writing a new 'topic sentence' for the top of that paragraph. You may have four important reasons why the sky is blue, so the topic sentence could be, *There are four key reasons why the sky is blue.* The existing sentences remain, but they become supporting sentences.

This test can show you the underlying structure of your writing – the bones and the flesh. This allows you to make informed decisions about whether your paragraph structure is working well, or whether you need to strengthen it. (The test is also useful when applied to other people's writing, particularly when you are trying to work out why a piece does not appear to be working.)

TASK 19: Yellow marker test. Do the yellow marker test on your own work. Can you strengthen the structure? If so, do so.

The third test of structure does not really look at a macro-editing issue, but it is a simple and elegant test that fits in well with the previous two. The first words of a piece of writing are vital because they will form the reader's first impression, so it makes sense that they should have as much impact as possible (or at least not be boring). In the following sentence, the first six words are dull, a kind of throat clearing: *Following extensive discussions by the policy sub-committee of the Trust, it was decided that the hospital will re-open.* Turn it around, so that the first sentence starts with the more interesting words: *The hospital will re-open, the policy sub-committee of the Trust has decided after extensive discussions.*

TASK 20: First-six-words test. Now write down the first six words ONLY of your piece of writing. If they are dull, rewrite the sentence.

QUESTION 5: IS THE TONE APPROPRIATE?

By tone I mean the overall impression that your writing is giving. Are you using the tone of the public bar when you should be using that of the courtroom, or the tone of a professional when you are writing for a patient? Are you being needlessly pompous, or are you being clear and simple when you actually need to be pompous (in a submission to government for instance)?

There is an excellent way of testing for tone: the Gunning Fog test. It was developed in the 1940s by Professor Gunning, an American journalism professor, as part of the attempt to measure 'reading age'. Over the years it has become clear that it can not really do this, but what remain particularly useful are (a) its relative simplicity, and (b) its capacity to measure the length of sentences and the length of words and construct out of these an index that allows us to compare various pieces of writing.

GUNNING FOG TEST

Step one: Take a section of text (there is no reason why you shouldn't start at the beginning) and count up to about 100 words. I say 'about' because your selection needs to end at a full stop.

Step two: Calculate the average sentence length by dividing 100 by the number of sentences in the passage chosen.

Step three: Count the number of words with three or more syllables. This figure gives you the number of difficult words. Don't count:
- proper nouns, e.g. Winchester, Manchester
- combinations of easy words, like 'photocopy'
- verbs that become three syllables when you add 'es', 'ing', 'ed' (e.g. 'committed').

Step four: Add the average sentence length (as calculated in step two) to the number of difficult words (as calculated in step three).

Step five: Multiply the total in step four by 0.4 to get the reading score.

Example one: An action group was formed within the *community* by the more *vociferous individuals* in 2006, which included local *councillors*, with the expressed object of campaigning for a local *surgery*. Following a variety of *incongruous* and *inconsequential* moves, the group *eventually* approached the medical *practices* whose current *responsibilities* included the village of Dudgeham.

Inexplicably the Patients Action Group did not *communicate* with the *committee* and, therefore, the latter was not afforded the *opportunity* to explain the *parameters* of *provision* for a *surgery* for GPs nor the limited powers at their *disposal* for *negatively* controlling the *distribution* of *medical* manpower within any given *geographical locality*.

Example two: Local *councillors* and others formed an action group to campaign for a local *surgery*. They approached the doctors who covered the village. The Patients Action Group did not speak to the PCT, which therefore could not explain the rules for providing a GP *surgery* or its limited powers of controlling where GPs work.

In September 2006 Dr Prodder asked if his practice could open a branch *surgery* in Dudgeham. Our practice premises *manager* inspected the proposed site and decided that, with some *internal* changes, it would be *suitable*. The PCT gave outline *approval*.

	Example one	Example two
Sentence length	33	17
No. of long words	23	8
Total	56	25
Reading score	22.4	10

Sample scores:

Airport novels	8–10
Tabloid newspapers	10–12
Middlebrow newspapers	12–14
Medical journals	14–16
Obscure journals	16–18
Insurance policies	18–20
An early NICE document	22

The important thing about the Fog score is not whether it is high or low, but whether it is (in your judgment as the writer) *appropriate* to your target audience. If you are writing for a *Sun* reader, then your score should be 8–10. If you are writing for a middlebrow newspaper or a professional newspaper, it should be 12–14. If you are writing for an academic journal, it should be 14–18. If your score is not in the appropriate range, that doesn't mean that you should immediately try to manipulate it; but you should consider whether you need to change the tone of your writing, for instance by using shorter sentences or simpler alternatives to the words you have chosen.

I once came across an experienced hospital manager who routinely answered complaints as part of his job. I found that when he received a letter with a Fog score of 9 he would reply at about 9; when he received a letter with a Fog score of 15 he would reply at about 15. He had no idea he was doing this, but it showed that over the years he had developed his skills to such an extent that he was automatically responding to his target audience in the language they were using. (This also shows, incidentally, the value of writing for one audience at a time: if you are writing for several, such targeting is not possible.)

DISCUSSION POINT: Simple or simplistic?
One of the things that quickly became obvious in my writing courses is that many professional people (particularly doctors) feel a piece of writing with a low score is vulgar ('Janet and John' or 'Mickey Mouse' is how they described it). This makes writing for those professional groups very difficult. Do you make the writing complicated in order to meet their expectations, even though this makes it less likely that they will read and understand it? Or do you keep it simple, knowing that they will understand the message, but probably think little of the writer? There is probably no easy answer here, though you should make a decision on the tone you will use before you start writing, and try to keep to it.

TASK 21: Do the Gunning Fog test on the piece of writing you are working on. Is it appropriate for the audience?

(a) Number of sentences

(b) Average sentence length

(c) Number of long words

(d) Add (b) and (c)

(e) Multiply by 0.4 to get your Fog score

A NOTE ON BALANCED FEEDBACK

These five questions – message, market, evidence, structure and tone – provide a good checklist for deciding whether your writing is good enough to 'publish' (i.e. send to the target audience). They also provide an excellent framework for giving – and getting – *balanced feedback*. Instead of going through a text line by line, making changes as you go, you could read the whole work, sit back – and then ask the five questions. Work out what has been done well, and what needs further work.

Examples of balanced feedback

▌ 'Your message seems to be that we need £500,000 to set up a new banana smoking clinic. This is a good message, and I think you are right to put this in a report to the chief executive. You make the case for what you say. The language is nice and simple. It seems a little long at 5,000 words, and it might be easier for the chief executive to digest if it were shorter.'

▌ 'Your message seems to be that bananas will help people who want to give up smoking. This is a new and important message and I think it is right for the British Journal of Smoking Cessation. The language is fine for a journal article. I see that you have six paragraphs in the introduction and only three in the discussion: you should look at the journal carefully to see what they do, but I suspect that you need to transfer some information from the introduction to the discussion.'

TASK 22: Give yourself balanced feedback on your own piece of writing, using the following main headings:

Message

Market

Evidence

Structure

Tone

WHAT YOU CAN NOW DO

▮ Apply five 'macro-editing' questions to a piece of writing.
▮ Make a decision on the basis of those five questions as to whether your writing is good enough to move forward for final polishing.
▮ Use these five questions to give balanced feedback to yourself and others.

Rewriting – sweat the details

Now is the time to get the details right – the *micro-editing*. Failure to do so will not destroy the writing in the way that failure to sort out the macro-issues will, but it could damage your credibility, make you a laughing stock – and distract readers from the message. Besides, you have a duty to your readers to get things as accurate as possible.

This is hard work and may hurt. Don't try doing everything at once. You may find it useful to print out the document, and go through your manuscript looking at the following:

- facts
- omissions
- grammar
- punctuation
- spelling
- style.

After a while, you should be able to do some or all of these functions at the same time, but for the purpose of this exercise I recommend you do them one by one.

1 FACTS

Go back to your notes or original data to check that everything you have written is accurate. If you have numbers, recalculate them. If you have direct quotations, make sure they are word-for-word. Do not take any short cuts and be particularly careful with the following:

■ Names and titles: People get very offended if you get these wrong, and there are many pitfalls, such as Ann and Anne and Brown and Browne, not to mention Mc and Mac. Calling someone a *deputy assistant* instead of an *assistant deputy* is likely to be a poor career move.

■ Dosages: A decimal point moving sideways could decimate populations.

> TASK 23: Go through what you have written sentence by sentence, asking yourself if you KNOW that everything you have written (names, details etc.) is accurate. If you are doubtful, go back and check.

If your writing is going to have references, put them in now. The purpose of references is not to display how many of them you know (or can find electronically), but to support the facts. Go through your text sentence by sentence, and work out which statements need to be supported. Be rigorous: some studies of academic journals have revealed that as many as two-thirds of references are wrong, with both citation errors (they can't be found where they are said to be), and quotation errors (once you get to them, they are saying something different). This is clearly unacceptable.

> TASK 24: If your target audience is expecting references, go through the writing sentence by sentence, and add references where needed.

2 OMISSIONS

Scan your notes. Make sure you haven't left out anything vital. If you think you have, bear in mind that if you add something, you might have to take something away.

> TASK 25: Go through your original notes and identify anything that should be included. Add it where appropriate, and make cuts if necessary.

3 SPELLING

Misspelling a word can lead to ambiguity: *we need a new role* is not the same as *we need a new roll* (or even *we knead a new roll*). Spell-checks have made it easier to avoid errors, but be alert for good words in the wrong place, such as the *peach and quiet* I managed to spot in a not-so-early draft of this book. (Or, if you want to ruin Sheikhspeare: *Two bee whore knot two bee, that is the quest shun/Weather tease no blur in the mined . . .*) Ask a friend, colleague or lover to proofread for you (*see* next session), but be careful not to engage in literary or philosophical debate.

4 GRAMMAR

When you are confident about the spelling, read through for grammatical problems. You may not know many of the rules (few people do nowadays), but applying common sense will help. *Please make an appointment with the secretary for the doctor* is clear. *Please make an appointment for the doctor with the secretary* could mean the same thing, or it could mean the doctor wants to see the secretary – or it could mean that you should book only with the doctor with a secretary. It gets confusing, which is why you have to get it right.

Use aids (like computer programs – and reference books!), and don't be afraid to delegate. Some people have an aptitude for grammar (and learnt it at school), so ask them for help. The grammar-check on Microsoft Word can also be helpful, though you must not blindly accept everything it recommends.

A word of warning, however: there are some so-called 'grammatical rules' that, when you look them up, turn out not to be rules at all, but matters of style. That doesn't stop your critics from treating you as an uneducated idiot. The main so-called rules are:

▌ do not start a sentence with *And* or *But* (as in: *But we were told not to*)

▌ do not split an infinitive (as in: *to boldly go*)

▌ do not end a sentence with a preposition (as in: *let us go up*).

The experts now consider these acceptable.

> TASK 26: Check your work for grammatical errors.

5 PUNCTUATION

Punctuation is also important. These tiny little marks can sometimes make a terrific difference, as Lynne Truss has made clear with her widely quoted book title *Eats, shoots and leaves*. If you are unsure about punctuation, you should again consider enlisting the help of friend, colleague or lover. If you want to brush up on your own punctuation skills, some advice is provided in Part 4, List 4, p. 112.

> TASK 27: Make sure that there are no major punctuation errors.

> DISCUSSION POINT: Pompous initial capitals
>
> Health professionals often overuse initial capital letters. Thus: *It is advised that patients make an appointment for the Doctor with the Nurse or the Departmental Secretary.* There are several problems with this. First, it is not grammatical: these words are being used as common nouns, not proper nouns, so don't need an initial capital. Second, it is typographically ugly and can be difficult to read. Third, and most important, it appears to be used in order to denote status. If we have *Doctors, Nurses* and *Departmental Secretaries,* we should also have *Patients* (and *Window Cleaners*), but we don't. The best solution is to use initial capitals sparingly. Proper nouns (a place or name like *Manchester* or the *Department of Psychology at the University of Manchester* or the *Sound of Music*) take an initial capital because they are unique. But individually and thereafter it should be the *department, psychology, university, doctor, sound and music.*

> TASK 28: Take out any pompous initial capitals.

6 STYLE

Style is always a problem, partly because no one seems to agree on what good style is, but also because many of us were led as children to believe that it reflected our abilities and even our personality. So it can become tense: when people criticise our style we feel they are criticising us.

First we need a sensible definition. Our model of effective writing (Session 2) leads us towards the following:

> A good style involves choosing words and constructing sentences in such a way that our writing is likely to get the message across to the target audience.

In other words, style should be reader-related, not author-related. Its purpose should not be to impress but to meet the needs and expectations of the target audience. A good stylist can write for the *Sun* in the morning (*Soup-a-scam!*), the *Telegraph* in the afternoon (*Too many cooks spoil the broth*), and knock out a few thousand words for a PhD thesis in the evening (*The evidence therefore suggests that a surfeit of catering operatives impacts negatively on liquidised nourishment*).

My advice is three-fold.
(i) Make an assessment of the kind of style that your audience will be comfortable with.

If you are not familiar with your target audience, you need to do some research. Consider what they read and what they don't read. Do a Gunning Fog test to assess the appropriate tone.

(ii) Keep your writing as clear as possible, without upsetting your target audience.

Writers who have commented on writing – such as George Orwell, Somerset Maugham, William Strunk and Keith Waterhouse – have long agreed that keeping things as simple as possible is the key to a good style. The main principles are:

▍ keep sentences short: four or five sentences per every 100 words
▍ use the active: *We have shown* rather than *it was shown*
▍ prefer simple words: *shown* rather than *demonstrated*
▍ make every word count: *now* rather than *at this present time*.

For those who have the time, energy and inclination, matters of style are explained more fully in Part 4.

How to polish your style

~~There are significant advantages when effective written~~
Good writing should be
~~communications are~~ rooted in clear thought~~,~~processes. ~~Such analyses~~
                    simply   *speaking to the*
It should be expressed ~~with~~ simplicity, as if the reader~~,~~ ~~was being~~
                              Avoid   *Prefer*
~~personally addressed.~~ Passive and negative sentences~~,~~ ~~should be~~
                                   simple and familiar
~~avoided like the plague. Rather than employing~~ words~~,~~ whose

~~prevailing characteristics are length and pomposity, simplicity and~~
                        Strike out
~~familiarity are preferred.~~ Redundant words should ~~be deleted~~ and
                              focus on
avoid clichés~~,~~~~avoided. It is generally considered that~~ people, objects and the

actions that relate them~~,~~~~should be the prime focus for your written~~

~~communication activities.~~

(iii) Don't spend too much time on style at this stage.
This advice may surprise you. But other people (such as colleagues, co-authors and supervisors) are about to review your writing, which generally means playing about with the style. So it is hardly worth investing much of your time, skill and ego on style at this stage. Save your energies for later, when you will have to make sense of the various stylistic suggestions from others.

DISCUSSION POINT: 'We're devaluing the language'

A common argument, particularly (but not exclusively) from those with a traditional (i.e. expensive) education, is that keeping things simple wastes the wealth and depth of the English language. 'We have so many wonderful words in the English language,' they say. 'Surely we should use them all?' Well, yes, up to a point. But the trick is to use them when they are appropriate, not just because they are there. The important thing is not to use a long and unfamiliar word when a short and familiar one will do.

TASK 29: Do a quick tidy-up of your manuscript so that it can be read clearly.

DEBATE DISCUSSION POINT: Political correctness

Not long ago, the word went out on training courses that the term *brainstorm* was forbidden on the grounds that it offended people with epilepsy. A year or so later, the word went round again that the groups representing those with epilepsy said this was nonsense and they were not offended. Such incidents – whether true or urban myth – go some way to explaining the concern in some quarters that 'political correctness' is ruining the English language.

Words are important in defining our culture, and we do need to be careful which ones we use, steering clear not just of sexist and racist ones, but of any likely to cause unnecessary offence. But the danger is that we take this too far, worry about it too much and end up saying too little. The best approach is to not worry about 'political correctness' at all as you write the first (and private) draft. When you rewrite it, however, look over it with a view to making sure you are not going to offend needlessly.

WHAT YOU CAN NOW DO

- Improve the quality of a piece of writing by applying four micro-editing questions.
- Know what makes a good style – and how to achieve it.

Getting others to help (not hinder)

Your troubles are nearly over. Having sweated to get your writing to a position where you think it is likely to work, you now have to pass your beautiful creation to others. Not only will they have different agendas (remember the *false feedback loop*, Session 3), but they will also have spent far less time thinking about the writing than you have. Don't be intimidated.

If you hand out a pile of papers and ask for 'Comments, please', don't complain when it comes back full of red marks. You need to be specific about what you want people to do, and you should not simply accept what they say. Consider each proposed change against this question: will it help my writing get across that brick wall to the target audience?

1 VOLUNTEERS

First, you may wish to show your writing to people informally. Here are some people to try, and how to brief them.

▌ Your spouse or partner: Show them your work if you can, because they are good at asking basic questions and spotting errors that you no longer see because you put them there in the first place, e.g. *I lost a stone in a wee*, or *The residents much enjoyed playing carpet bowels*. If you have no partner, find someone who enjoys being picky.
Brief to partner: Can you find any stupid errors in here?

■ A colleague: They should know about the topic, so will be able to point out if you have left out anything of major importance, or if your argument has gaping holes.
Brief to colleague: Can you see any major pitfalls in here?
■ A reader: It is vital to find someone who is typical of your target audience to see (a) whether they understand what you have written and (b) whether they find it interesting.
Brief to reader: Can you tell me if you understand this? Do you find it interesting?

At this stage you are in control. If you disagree with what they say, you can ignore their comments. You do need to be diplomatic, though: if you ignore everything they say all the time, they will eventually become demotivated and stop helping.

> TASK 30: Take the piece you have written and try it on three different people, giving each a different brief.

2 BOSSES

These could be your line managers, or they could be people who have some power over you (like co-authors whose signatures you need before you submit an article). Here you have to be more careful – and this is where your upward management skills come into effect.

You should already have discussed the brief with your boss(es) (*see* Session 3). If you have managed to agree over message, market and pay-off, you could remind them of that, and try to steer them on to other tasks, such as whether your writing risks political or legal repercussions.

When their comments come back, you need to do a triage. Some of your boss's comments will be extremely useful (and likely to help your writing cross that brick wall). In such cases, thank them profusely. Other comments (almost certainly the majority) will not make any real difference to whether your message gets across, but if you're smart you will thank the boss for their contribution, and make the changes. (Some alpha-persons say they will ignore these comments, but that's a high-risk approach.)

Finally, there are the comments that, in your opinion, will ruin all your good work and ensure that your message crashes into the brick wall and is lost forever. You need to negotiate. Remind your boss of the fantastic contribution they have already made, and then provide evidence for why you don't like the latest suggestion. ('I have looked at the last five reports that got funding. None of them are longer than three sides of A4, and they all use very short words.') But stress that the decision is theirs: 'What do *you* think we should do?'

In short, the principles are:

▮ lose the battles that aren't important
▮ make everything evidence-based
▮ do not turn it into a power struggle.

> TASK 31: Show your draft to your boss (or co-author). Go through the comments, working out which ones you need to negotiate over. Do so.

One common problem is getting people to process the writing. Again, referring back to the brief and reminding them that you have an agreed deadline may be of some help. It may sometimes be necessary to give people a polite ultimatum. Sometimes you can threaten to take their name out of the document, but often you will just have to wait. It might be worth instituting a paper trail so that it is clear who is holding things up.

3 THE WIDER WORLD

There is little more pleasurable than sending off a piece of writing, and relaxing. Of course, there is probably going to be some choppy water ahead: after all, writing involves committing yourself (usually in black and white), and this will attract comments. This can be dispiriting (which is often the intention of the critics anyway) but remember that effective writing is judged on whether it succeeds in its purpose, and not on whether every single detail is unimpeachable. And always remember that, whenever someone criticises what you have written, it does mean you have succeeded in making them read it!

WHAT YOU CAN NOW DO

▌ Use the skills and knowledge of other people to improve your manuscript.

▌ Use the skills and knowledge of your bosses and co-authors to improve the manuscript, and resist suggestions that will make it worse.

Epilogue: Bringing it all together

Congratulations. You have made it to the end of the workbook, and at the same time worked up a piece of writing. While I don't expect you to use all the suggestions in this book for everything you write, I hope that you have acquired some useful tricks and techniques. More importantly, I hope that you are now able to look on writing in a slightly different – and more relaxed – way. I also hope that you have acquired greater confidence in your own abilities.

TASK 32: Go back to Task 4, where you were asked to write down three goals. Did you achieve them?

Task 32 (*continued*)

How do you make sure that you keep these gains? First, I recommend that in a month or two you return to this book and look at Part 2. The purpose is to help you find out where you might still be having problems, and to suggest what might be going wrong – and what further action you might take. On a still longer time frame, you might wish to consult the fourth and final part, which is intended to stimulate your interest in matters of grammar and style.

TIPS FOR SOME TOP BOOKS

I said earlier I wouldn't give a *long* list of reading, but for those who wish to take their exploration of writing a little further, here is an extremely biased *short* list of some of my favourite books:

- *The Elements of Style* by William Strunk and EB White, Allyn and Bacon, 1999. This is a much reprinted classic, with excellent advice on how to develop an effective writing style.
- *On Writing: a memoir of the craft* by Stephen King, New English Library, 2001. Although King writes fiction, he offers revealing insights on the process of writing, plus a list of 'must read' books from Ruth Rendell to Graham Greene.
- *Medical Writing: a prescription for clarity*, Neville Goodman and Martin Edwards, Cambridge University Press, 2006. This is a merciless attack on current medical writing, plus sensible advice on how to do better.
- *The King's English: a guide to modern usage* by Kingsley Amis, HarperCollins, 1997. This book is a sensible look at grammar and style, and a little livelier than some of the others.
- *Advice to Writers: a compendium of quotes, anecdotes, and writerly wisdom from a dazzling array of literary lights* compiled by Jon Winokur, Pavilion Books, 1999. Winokur has collected some wonderful pieces of advice, from Somerset Maugham's 'A good style should show no sign of effort' to TS Eliot's 'Whatever you do ... avoid piles.'
- *How Not to Write: simple guidelines for the grammatically perplexed*, Terence Denman, Piatkus Books, 2005. Denman's book is a sensible and readable guide to some of the vagaries of the English language.

The most valuable way forward, of course, is continuing to write. As I mentioned earlier, I give no guarantee that you will always write without pain. But your skills should continue to grow, and as they do you will acquire a powerful tool.

As a final note, I would like to thank all those who read an early version of this book and gave invaluable feedback: in particular Jane Cass, Steve Coveney, Deborah Kay, Liz Easterbrook, Andrew Ascroft, and David Herne, all from Central Lancashire PCT, and Ruth Milton. I would like to thank Jane Donovan, Wynford Hicks, Neville Goodman, Jim and Liz Wager, and Harvey Marcovitch for their help with various lists in Part 4. Nigel Grant was particularly kind and helpful in giving detailed comments on the whole of this section. I would also like to thank those at Radcliffe Publishing for giving me the chance to write another book. Shelley Hemming did a superb editing job, adding consistency to the whole, and perceptively querying some of my long-held assumptions. I would like to thank Barbara, who had to endure the spousal suffering (and proofreading) all over again. Finally, I would like to thank all those who came on my courses: I learnt far more from them than they did from me.

TASK 33: Write down three possible ways of celebrating the fact that you have just completed your writing assignment. Then choose one of them and do it.

Part 2

After-sales service

I would love to say that all your writing problems will melt away as soon as you have completed this workbook, but that won't happen. There will be gains, but there will also be setbacks, such as difficulties adapting to a new technique, regression into old habits or simply confusion. This is natural.

I suggest that, some 10 or so weeks after you have completed the 10-step programme that makes up Part 1 of this book, you assess your progress. Go through the following questionnaire, which is virtually the same as the one you did at the start of the workbook. Without referring to your original answers, tick those statements that apply to you now.

- ☐ 1. I do not have enough time to write
- ☐ 2. I have too many ideas
- ☐ 3. I find it difficult to write for different types of audiences
- ☐ 4. I find it difficult to stop researching
- ☐ 5. I tend to write too much – or too little
- ☐ 6. I often get stuck during a writing project
- ☐ 7. I spend too much time rewriting
- ☐ 8. My writing tends to come back full of changes* from other people
- ☐ 9. I do not know what is meant by 'good writing'
- ☐ 10. I would like to be able to write more easily

Note: changes, not corrections

1 I do not have enough time to write

This one doesn't go away easily. Writing takes a lot of time, and we tend to underestimate how much.

One solution is to become more efficient. If you think this is your way forward, write down how long you think your next major piece should take. Break it down into the various stages (e.g. 10 minutes for setting the brief; 15 minutes for planning; 30 minutes for writing; 60 minutes for rewriting). When you come to write it, record how much time you *actually* take. This should show you what you are doing (not just what you think you are doing) and where you could save time.

If you find you are spending too much time planning, there is probably not much you can do. You could consider making a better use of 'down time' – lying in bed or the bath, travelling in the bus, having a quiet coffee. But the thinking process can't, and shouldn't, be rushed. You might find, however, that you get better and quicker at it over time.

If you are taking too much time writing your first draft, you will have strayed (deliberately or not) from the technique of free writing (page 49). I appreciate that it's not for everyone, but I recommend that you try it at least one more time: set yourself 10 or 15 minutes and, with just your plan in front of you, start writing. If you use this technique, you will certainly be able to write your draft more quickly – and you will probably have less to cut once you have written it.

If your problem is endless rewriting, at your behest or at the behest of others, then see the discussions on questions 7 and 8 below.

Overall, a sensible use of deadlines is particularly helpful; some might say essential. If they are not imposed on you, impose them on yourself. Don't just set one end-point, have several interim deadlines for completing key tasks along the way. Make these deadlines realistic: not so near that you can't help but break them, and not so far away that they fall off your agenda and become overtaken by other things. Discipline yourself to keeping them. This will help you keep up the momentum, and also give you a firm cut-off point. If you persist in breaking deadlines, look for an underlying reason, such as over-optimistic timings, lack of commitment or an unconscious desire to keep people waiting. When you understand why you are breaking these deadlines, you should be able to change your habits (or attitude!).

Finally, ask whether your problem is simply that you are having to write too much. If so, you have two alternatives: say no, or delegate to someone else. One of the best ways of writing well is to limit the amount of writing you do. This suggestion may sound drastic, but how often could a long interchange of emails be replaced by a quick telephone call?

ACTIVITIES

- Revisit Sessions 4–7.
- Analyse your writing processes to see where you could be more efficient.
- Identify areas of 'down time' you could profitably use to ruminate.
- Have one more go at free writing. You could even try writing the draft with your computer screen turned off.
- Go on a course (or read a book) on time management.
- Review the way you are setting – and keeping – deadlines.
- Review what you have to write, and come up with one piece that you need not do yourself.
- Practise saying no.

2 I have too many ideas

Don't knock ideas; they are extremely useful and many people find they don't come along often enough. If you have plenty of them you should be pleased. Don't waste them; make sure you have a good way of recording them, either electronically or by using a good old-fashioned notebook. This will put them on hold while you do other things – such as writing.

However, if you find that new ideas and information keep bubbling to the surface and limiting your ability to follow through the ones you already have, try to be focused. The time for focusing is when you define the message (page 22). Make sure it is tightly written: use specific language; make it short enough to contain one idea only; and include a verb, which will pin you down on exactly what you want to say.

Once you are satisfied with your message, move on swiftly. The faster you move, the less chance you will allow yourself to have second thoughts. You can have these later, in their proper place, which is in the rewriting stage, but do not allow them to intrude before then. (Which takes us back to the usefulness of a notebook.)

ACTIVITIES

▌ Revisit Session 4.
▌ Carry a notebook to capture your brilliant ideas.
▌ Check whether the message of a current or imminent piece of writing is sufficiently focused; if not, amend.
▌ Take your next piece of writing from message to first draft without doing any more research.

3 I find it difficult to write for different types of audiences

If your problem is that you find it difficult to write for an unfamiliar audience (or, even worse, that an unfamiliar audience is finding it difficult to understand what you are writing), you need to do some market research. Think about your target audience. What publications are they likely to read regularly? What kind of other reading are they likely to do? What, if anything, have they written? If you can get hold of their writing, analyse it by applying some of the tests covered in Session 8, such as the yellow marker test (page 53) and the Gunning Fog test (page 55). Look at the length and complexity of their sentences and words. Speak to representatives of your target audience. Show them something you have written. Do they understand it? Do they find it interesting? The more you get to know your target audiences, the easier you will find it to write for them.

This works well when you are writing for one audience at a time, but the constant pressure to write for several is less easy to address. It is a flawed approach: each of these audiences will have different requirements, and you will not be able to meet them all; in fact, communicating well to some may antagonise others. The only solution is to focus on one audience at a time; all else is compromise. If you want to communicate to other audiences, you should do so by targeting them directly with a separate document (e.g. report, executive summary, press release, letter) for each (*see* layering, page 17).

Do not be overly influenced by others. If your colleagues or your boss do not like what you have written, remember that it is not aimed at them.

ACTIVITIES

▌ Revisit Session 3.
▌ Take a piece of writing you had trouble with, and ask yourself if you really were writing for one specific audience.
▌ Take the same piece of writing and ask if you could have 'layered' it (i.e. written different versions for different audiences).
▌ Take a short passage you have written (or even a single sentence) and try to rewrite it for specific audiences (e.g. readers of the Sun, the Guardian, The Times, romantic novels, scientific papers, Department of Health reports).
▌ Ask one or two members from your target audience to read what you have written and underline anything they find difficult or impossible to understand – or just boring.
▌ Ask a colleague (or your boss) to do the same, and see whether they are highlighting the same things. (If not, you have an excellent example of the false feedback loop in action.)

4 I find it difficult to stop researching

There usually comes a tipping point when the amount of information you have collected is enough to enable you to define a message and start to plan your writing. The difficult part is to recognise when this point arrives, as it often comes earlier than you might think.

Two techniques are of use. The first is to keep trying out possible messages as you do the research (or even before). They will probably evolve and change in the early stages, but there will come a time when the message stops evolving. That signals the time to stop researching and start working up the writing. The second technique is to set a deadline for putting away the research and starting to define the brief. This will give you a cutoff point that will concentrate the mind wonderfully.

Some people worry that they will leave out data or information or parts of an argument. Of course you will leave something out, because that is the point of writing: it forces you to make selections and order your information. But the omissions are unlikely to be crucial, and anyway, the planning and rewriting stages should allow you to identify *major* shortcomings or omissions, and you will have plenty of time to rectify them.

ACTIVITIES
▌ Revisit Sessions 4 and 5.
▌ As you research a piece of writing, keep experimenting with possible messages.
▌ Try setting a deadline after which you will not do any more research until the first draft is complete.

5 I tend to write too much – or too little
This should not still be happening. You should be working to a plan that enables you to write roughly the number of words required. If you are not working to a plan, you have only yourself to blame if you are writing too much or too little.

More probably, you are working to a plan but still not meeting the approximate length requirements. Several things could be going wrong. First, the plan could be inappropriate, i.e. have too many or too few paragraphs. Work out in advance how many paragraphs will be appropriate, and then plan for that number. It won't always be exact, but it shouldn't be far out.

Second, if your plan does have an appropriate number of paragraphs, but you are still writing too much or too little, you may have a problem with the length of your paragraphs. As a rough guide, you should have about five sentences, or 100–120 words, per paragraph. If you are writing your paragraphs as 'inverted triangles' starting with the topic sentence (page 41), you shouldn't have much difficulty in cutting out, or putting in, a sentence or two at the end of a paragraph.

A third possible problem is that although you have a plan of the right length, you ignore it as you write. The answer here is discipline – and free writing (*see* page 49). Keep focused as you write, and don't give yourself time to go off on tangents. If you feel you need to make a substantial change, then note it down and look at it when you come to rewriting. Don't change your plan as you write.

A final possibility is that you – or others – keep adding or subtracting paragraphs from your first draft. Be firm, with yourself and others: if anything goes in, something should come out, and (if you are under-writing) when anything goes out then something should go in.

ACTIVITIES

▌ Revisit Sessions 6 and 7.

▌ Look at your plan, and if it is too long (or too short), write a new plan that will help give the required length.

▌ Take a message, and try drafting different plans for different sizes (e.g. three paragraphs, seven paragraphs, 14 paragraphs).

▌ Take something you have written and try shortening it (or lengthening it) by taking out (or putting in) sentences at the end of each paragraph.

▌ Have another go at free writing, and see if that enables you to keep to your plan.

6 I often get stuck during a writing project

If you are still suffering from writer's block, you need to identify where in the process you are getting stuck.

If you are finding it hard to get started, then, paradoxically, you need to slow down. The most likely reason is that you are trying to write before you are ready. Go back to the beginning of the process and make sure that you are absolutely clear about the following: the message you want to convey (one sentence only, with a verb), the target audience at whom you are aiming (one only) and the pay-off (achievable and measurable). If you haven't written a brief (page 21), do so. If you have, then look at it carefully. Is it specific enough? Is it what you want to do? Is it what others want you to do? Is there a difference between these two? Above all, don't panic and don't rush. Work out carefully what you are doing, and once that is clear, the writing task becomes straightforward.

If you are bogged down in the middle of a piece of writing, you have probably lost focus. Your brief may have been too baggy, or something may have come up to raise serious questions (it happens). Don't plough on regardless. Take time to go back to the beginning, examine your brief, and see whether you need to change it. Don't get discouraged if you do: it will probably take less time than you think, and will almost certainly save you time in the long run.

Not all writer's block is caused by lack of focus. Sometimes it is simply a question of fatigue (and boredom). If this is happening to you, reconsider the writing process you have adopted. After three or four hours of writing, fatigue will almost certainly creep in. Instead, aim to write for relatively short bursts of time (10–30 minutes), and take plenty of breaks. The fresher you are, the fresher your writing will be.

ACTIVITIES
▌ Revisit Session 4.
▌ Determine at which stage you get blocked, and analyse the reasons.
▌ Look back at a brief you have given yourself and see whether it could have been tighter.
▌ Review your writing process to see whether you can reduce fatigue and boredom.

7 I spend too much time rewriting

How much rewriting is 'too much'? Some people resent having to rewrite at all, seeing it as an admission of failure. But it is a vital part of the whole writing process, and is the place where your early thoughts are turned into effective prose. And it's hard work (*see* 10 below).

Don't worry about spending time in the macro-editing stage. This is when you will be looking at the big issues (message, market, pay-off, structure and tone), and you need to get these right if your work is to have a chance of succeeding. You need to be thorough. However, if you keep having to make the same type of changes – such as *always* having to alter the message, or *always* having to restructure the writing – you may need to look at what you are doing (or not doing) earlier on. Perhaps you need to define the message more tightly or pay greater attention to your plans.

Micro-editing is another matter altogether. Careful work is needed, but there is often a temptation to waste time, generally by fiddling with the text. You might wish to divide the micro-editing into various stages (checking for facts, putting in references, checking for style, etc.) and do each on a paper printout rather than on screen. This avoids the danger of it turning into a kind of computer game, with rewards coming from the pleasure of zapping words and whizzing around sentences rather than making – and being able to see – solid progress. Making changes on paper will allow you to see what you are doing as a whole, and to compare what you have done at different stages. You should be able to see progress and, more importantly, recognise when the changes start to dry up, repeat themselves, or become less important. This should signal to you that it is time to move on to the next stage, and ask others to read what you have written.

The danger is that micro-editing becomes a displacement activity, caused by the fear of putting your writing into the public domain. Remember that you are trying to achieve a pay-off, not write a perfect piece of prose. It is still a work in progress, and you have time to set things right.

ACTIVITIES
❚ Revisit Sessions 8 and 9.
❚ Analyse where in the rewriting process you are taking too much time.
❚ Keep a note of what you are having to change in the macro-editing stage. If you are persistently having to change the same aspect, see whether you can forestall these problems by making changes to how you write.
❚ Keep a hard copy of each run-through as you micro-edit and look at the changes you are making: are they necessary?
❚ Consider doing a course on proofreading that will enable you to pick up errors.
❚ Buy and read a simple book on grammar.
❚ Ask someone else to do some 'guest micro-editing' of something you are writing, and then compare what each of you has done.

8 My writing tends to come back full of changes from other people

It almost always will, and that's not necessarily a reflection of your ability as a writer, or of what you have written. You should have noticed in the last few weeks that the writing culture in which you are working is characterised by a high degree of criticism, so critical comments are the norm.

But you should be able to reduce the number of comments. Try to get agreement over the main points (message, market and pay-off) before you start writing. For particularly sensitive pieces (or situations), you may want to have something in writing so that all can see when the specifications are being changed. Try to direct these critics to answering specific questions or performing specific tasks, such as confirming whether a piece of writing is likely to achieve the pay-off or identifying grammatical errors. You might also want to encourage balanced feedback, so that your critics can summarise not just what you are doing badly (or if you want to be more positive, 'what needs to be worked on'), but also what you are doing well.

A positive attitude at this stage is crucial. Remember these people are suggesting changes, not making 'corrections'. You have an opportunity to improve your writing, but you must be tough and confident. You are the expert in what you are writing.

ACTIVITIES
▌ Revisit Session 10.
▌ Read a book or do a course on negotiation skills.
▌ Read a book or do a course on assertiveness skills.
▌ Buy a standard and respected work like *Fowler's Modern English Usage* to help you back up your negotiations.
▌ Do a course on proofreading or plain English.

9 I do not know what is meant by 'good writing'

This should not be a problem. One of the most important messages in this workbook is that 'good writing' is determined by whether you succeed in what you set out to do. This outcome is not difficult to establish. Decide as you set the brief (page 21) how you can measure whether your writing has worked, and measure accordingly. Do not be sidetracked (or intimidated) when people attack your writing for any other reason.

If your writing achieves what it sets out to do, it is good enough. If you aspire to more than that, try evening classes in creative writing.

ACTIVITIES
▌ Revisit Session 3.
▌ Keep working out in advance what you think the pay-off (see page 27) should be.
▌ Look back at a couple of things you have written recently, and ask if your pay-off was achievable and measurable as well as desired.

10 I would like to be able to write more easily

I hope that you have not ticked this a second time around. Good writing requires pain, but it should now be more manageable. I hope that any pain is outweighed by the benefits you know you have achieved.

ACTIVITIES

▮ Write down five things you have achieved with your writing since you read this book, and ask if the pain was worth it.

▮ If you answer no, ask what implications there would be if you gave up writing altogether.

Part 3

Some points on design

Reading is visual. Thus, all the hard work in planning, writing and rewriting can be undone by a poor decision on design and layout. For the next few pages, I have written a mock job description for a writer, and then laid it out in different ways. Below is a commentary on what I have done and the effects that these decisions might have. You may wish to look at the different examples first and write down a quick reaction (one word will do).

1   This is laid out reasonably enough. The typeface is well known (Times New Roman) and a readable size (12 point). But it is dull, with no emphasis on the various levels of the writing.

2   Two decisions make this much more attractive and therefore reader-friendly. These are to use bullet points with the various lists, and to increase the spacing between lines (traditionally called leading because in the old days they literally used extra lines of lead between the lines of metal letters).

3   In this version I have used a contrasting type (Arial). It is a *sans serif* (the serifs being the little twiddly bits at the extremities of the letters), has a more modern feel, and is assumed to be easier to read on screen (because of its relative simplicity).

4   This one is similar to version 3 (above), but because this typeface looks large in 12 point, many prefer to bring it down to 11 point.

5   This has an old-fashioned look to it. The headings are both in bold and underscored, which is considered unnecessary these days. Indeed, underscoring is rarely used now. Also, there is a profusion of pointless initial capital letters within the copy.

6   This is clear, though unexciting. There is good spacing between the lines, and differentiation between the title (in 16 point bold, but not underscored) and the headings (in bold).

7 This introduces two typefaces, one for the bulk of the article (the body copy) and the other for the titles and headings (display type). This looks attractive, and introduces a little personality.

8 This is an example of polyfontophilia – the love of many fonts. The overall impression is at best disorganised, at worst well outside the norm. It is also difficult to read (particularly the section in italics).

9 This looks mean-spirited. The margins are too narrow, which makes the copy look cramped (rather than framed in a reasonable bit of white space). And the narrow leading seems unnecessary, since there is plenty of room on the page for more space between the lines.

10 The type size is too large (14 point) and gives the impression that the author is shouting. The lack of bullet points doesn't help either.

1 JOB DESCRIPTION: WRITER

Purpose of role
To put across information, ideas and emotion from one person to
one or more others in order to meet a specific goal

Key responsibilities
To accept from another, or define oneself, a piece of information,
idea or emotion that needs transmitting in written form from one
person to another
To collect information from a number of sources – written,
electronic, spoken, etc.
To assess the information and from it make a judgment on a
message
To define the audience
To define the pay-off
To select from the information gathered data that will support the
message
To formulate an appropriate plan
To write the requisite number of words according to this plan
To revise the first draft according to macro-editing and micro-
editing principles
To measure whether the writing has achieved the stated pay-off

Person specification
Excellent time-management skills, including the ability to make
and meet deadlines
Good negotiation skills
Skills in researching information and assessing reliability
Reasonable knowledge of English language and grammar
Familiarity with Microsoft Word
A cheery disposition and the ability to celebrate when appropriate

2 JOB DESCRIPTION: WRITER

Purpose of role
- To put across information, ideas and emotion from one person to one or more others in order to meet a specific goal

Key responsibilities
- To accept from another, or define oneself, a piece of information, idea or emotion that needs transmitting in written form from one person to another
- To collect information from a number of sources – written, electronic, spoken, etc.
- To assess the information and from it make a judgment on a message
- To define the audience
- To define the pay-off
- To select from the information gathered data that will support the message
- To formulate an appropriate plan
- To write the requisite number of words according to this plan
- To revise the first draft according to macro-editing and micro-editing principles
- To measure whether the writing has achieved the stated pay-off

Person specification
- Excellent time-management skills, including the ability to make and meet deadlines
- Good negotiation skills
- Skills in researching information and assessing reliability
- Reasonable knowledge of English language and grammar
- Familiarity with Microsoft Word
- A cheery disposition and the ability to celebrate when appropriate

3 JOB DESCRIPTION: WRITER

Purpose of role
• To put across information, ideas and emotion from one person to one or more others in order to meet a specific goal

Key responsibilities
• To accept from another, or define oneself, a piece of information, idea or emotion that needs transmitting in written form from one person to another
• To collect information from a number of sources – written, electronic, spoken, etc.
• To assess the information and from it make a judgment on a message
• To define the audience
• To define the pay-off
• To select from the information gathered data that will support the message
• To formulate an appropriate plan
• To write the requisite number of words according to this plan
• To revise the first draft according to macro-editing and micro-editing principles
• To measure whether the writing has achieved the stated pay-off

Person specification
• Excellent time-management skills, including the ability to make and meet deadlines
• Good negotiation skills
• Skills in researching information and assessing reliability
• Reasonable knowledge of English language and grammar
• Familiarity with Microsoft Word
• A cheery disposition and the ability to celebrate when appropriate

4 JOB DESCRIPTION: WRITER

Purpose of role
- To put across information, ideas and emotion from one person to one or more others in order to meet a specific goal

Key responsibilities
- To accept from another, or define oneself, a piece of information, idea or emotion that needs transmitting in written form from one person to another
- To collect information from a number of sources – written, electronic, spoken, etc.
- To assess the information and from it make a judgment on a message
- To define the audience
- To define the pay-off
- To select from the information gathered data that will support the message
- To formulate an appropriate plan
- To write the requisite number of words according to this plan
- To revise the first draft according to macro-editing and micro-editing principles
- To measure whether the writing has achieved the stated pay-off

Person specification
- Excellent time-management skills, including the ability to make and meet deadlines
- Good negotiation skills
- Skills in researching information and assessing reliability
- Reasonable knowledge of English language and grammar
- Familiarity with Microsoft Word
- A cheery disposition and the ability to celebrate when appropriate

5 Job Description: writer

PURPOSE OF ROLE
• To put across Information, Ideas and Emotion from one person to one or more others in order to meet a Specific Goal

KEY REPONSIBILITIES
• To accept from another, or define oneself, a piece of information, idea or emotion that needs transmitting in written form from one person to another
• To collect information from a number of Sources – Written, Electronic, Spoken, etc.
• To assess the Information and from it make a judgment on a Message
• To define the Audience
• To define the Pay-off
• To select from the Information gathered data that will support the Message
• To formulate an appropriate Plan
• To write the requisite number of words according to this Plan
• To revise the First Draft according to Macro-editing and Micro-editing principles
• To measure whether the writing has achieved the stated Pay-off

PERSON SPECIFICATION
• Excellent Time-management Skills, including the ability to make and meet Deadlines
• Good Negotiation Skills
• Skills in researching information and assessing reliability
• Reasonable knowledge of English language and grammar
• Familiarity with Microsoft Word
• A cheery Disposition and the ability to celebrate when appropriate

6 Job description: writer

Purpose of role
• To put across information, ideas and emotion from one person to one or more others in order to meet a specific goal

Key responsibilities
• To accept from another, or define oneself, a piece of information, idea or emotion that needs transmitting in written form from one person to another
• To collect information from a number of sources – written, electronic, spoken, etc.
• To assess the information and from it make a judgment on a message
• To define the audience
• To define the pay-off
• To select from the information gathered data that will support the message
• To formulate an appropriate plan
• To write the requisite number of words according to this plan
• To revise the first draft according to macro-editing and micro-editing principles
• To measure whether the writing has achieved the stated pay-off

Person specification
• Excellent time-management skills, including the ability to make and meet deadlines
• Good negotiation skills
• Skills in researching information and assessing reliability
• Reasonable knowledge of English language and grammar
• Familiarity with Microsoft Word
• A cheery disposition and the ability to celebrate when appropriate

7 Job Description: writer

Purpose of role
• To put across information, ideas and emotion from one person to one or more others in order to meet a specific goal

Key responsibilities
• To accept from another, or define oneself, a piece of information, idea or emotion that needs transmitting in written form from one person to another
• To collect information from a number of sources – written, electronic, spoken, etc.
• To assess the information and from it make a judgment on a message
• To define the audience
• To define the pay-off
• To select from the information gathered data that will support the message
• To formulate an appropriate plan
• To write the requisite number of words according to this plan
• To revise the first draft according to macro-editing and micro-editing principles
• To measure whether the writing has achieved the stated pay-off

Person specification
• Excellent time-management skills, including the ability to make and meet deadlines
• Good negotiation skills
• Skills in researching information and assessing reliability
• Reasonable knowledge of English language and grammar
• Familiarity with Microsoft Word
• A cheery disposition and the ability to celebrate when appropriate

8 Job Description: writer

Purpose of role
- **To put across information, ideas and emotion from one person to one or more others in order to meet a specific goal**

Key responsibilities
- *To accept from another, or define oneself, a piece of information, idea or emotion that needs transmitting in written form from one person to another*
- *To collect information from a number of sources – written, electronic, spoken, etc.*
- *To assess the information and from it make a judgment on a message*
- *To define the audience*
- *To define the pay-off*
- *To select from the information gathered data that will support the message*
- *To formulate an appropriate plan*
- *To write the requisite number of words according to this plan*
- *To measure whether the writing has achieved the stated pay-off*

Person specification
- **Excellent time-management skills, including the ability to make and meet deadlines**
- **Good negotiation skills**
- **Skills in researching information and assessing reliability**
- **Reasonable knowledge of English language and grammar**
- **Familiarity with Microsoft Word**
- **A cheery disposition and the ability to celebrate when appropriate**

9 Job Description: writer

Purpose of role
• To put across information, ideas and emotion from one person to one or more others in order to meet a specific goal

Key responsibilities
• To accept from another, or define oneself, a piece of information, idea or emotion that needs transmitting in written form from one person to another
• To collect information from a number of sources – written, electronic, spoken, etc.
• To assess the information and from it make a judgment on a message
• To define the audience
• To define the pay-off
• To select from the information gathered data that will support the message
• To formulate an appropriate plan
• To write the requisite number of words according to this plan
• To revise the first draft according to macro-editing and micro-editing principles
• To measure whether the writing has achieved the stated pay-off

Person specification
• Excellent time-management skills, including the ability to make and meet deadlines
• Good negotiation skills
• Skills in researching information and assessing reliability
• Reasonable knowledge of English language and grammar
• Familiarity with Microsoft Word
• A cheery disposition and the ability to celebrate when appropriate

10 Job Description: writer

PURPOSE OF ROLE

To put across information, ideas and emotion from one person to one or more others in order to meet a specific goal

KEY RESPONSIBILITIES

To accept from another, or define oneself, a piece of information, idea or emotion that needs transmitting in written form from one person to another

To collect information from a number of sources – written, electronic, spoken, etc.

To assess the information and from it make a judgment on a message

To define the audience

To define the pay-off

To select from the information gathered data that will support the message

To formulate an appropriate plan

To write the requisite number of words according to this plan

To revise the first draft according to macro-editing and micro-editing principles

To measure whether the writing has achieved the stated pay-off

PERSON SPECIFICATION

Excellent time-management skills, including the ability to make and meet deadlines

Good negotiation skills

Part 4

Lists for the very keen

The list of lists

MAIN SOURCES FOR THIS SECTION

Albert, Tim. *A–Z of Medical Writing*. London: BMJ Books; 2000.
Albert, Tim. *Medical Journalism: the writer's guide*. Oxford: Radcliffe; 1992.

Amis, Kingsley. *The King's English: a guide to modern usage*. London: HarperCollins; 1997.

Bryson, Bill. *The Penguin Dictionary of Troublesome Words*. Hammondsworth: Penguin Books; 1984.

Burchfield, RW, editor. *Fowler's Modern English Usage*. 3rd ed. Oxford: Oxford University Press; 1996.

Carr, Sarah. *Tackling NHS Jargon: getting the message across*. Oxford: Radcliffe; 2002.

Evans, Harold. *Newsman's English*. London: Heinemann; 1990.

Goodman, Neville, and Edwards, Martin. *Medical Writing: a prescription for clarity*. 3rd ed. Cambridge: Cambridge University Press; 2006.

Hicks, Wynford. *English for Journalists*. 2nd ed. London: Routledge; 1998.

Howard, Godfrey. *The Good English Guide*. London: Macmillan; 1993.

Mayes, Ian. *Corrections and Clarifications*. London: Guardian Newspapers Ltd; 2000.

Strunk, William Jr, and White, EB. *The Elements of Style*. 4th ed. Boston: Allyn and Bacon; 1999.

Truss, Lynne. *Eats, Shoots and Leaves: the zero tolerance approach to punctuation*. London: Profile Books; 2003.

Winokur, John. *Advice to Writers: a compendium of quotes, anecdotes, and writerly wisdom from a dazzling array of literary lights*. London: Pavilion Books; 1999.

The parts of speech

Different kinds of words have different functions, and each kind has its own technical name. Does it help to know these names? Probably, if only to avoid being intimidated by those who think they do.

Nouns: The thing words: *desk, syringe, calculator, orange* (the fruit not the colour). Sometimes they are *abstract nouns,* because you can't see them – as in *faith, hope, ambition.* You can also have *proper nouns* (specific names) *such as Cocklehaven, Crohn* and *February*; and *collective nouns* for groups of things (department, committee, team).

Pronouns: Used instead of names to avoid repetition. *I, he, she* and *it* (subject); *me, him, her* and *it* (object): He *saw the orange.* She *took* it *off the desk and gave* it *to* him.

Adjectives: the words that 'qualify' the noun (add precision, interest, etc.). Examples are *the* ancient *hospital, the* scented *orange,* and *the* tidy *desk.*

Verbs: The action words (*doing, having, being*) that turn phrases into sentences: *The orange* rolled *across the desk and* fell *on the floor.*

Adverbs: The words that qualify (add precision, interest, etc.) to verbs, adjectives or other adverbs. They often end with a 'ly': *speedily, unwillingly, happily.* As in: *The clinical psychologist jumped* happily *into bed and slept* noisily.

Prepositions: These link a noun or phrase to another noun or phrase. This can be a difficult area (*see* Tricky Bit below). *I took a cup of coffee* to *the awakening psychologist.*

Conjunctions: Linking words, such as *and, but, or* and *if. I will go if you will.* Contrary to what people might tell you, it is acceptable to start a sentence with a conjunction.

TRICKY BIT: PREPOSITIONS

For small words, prepositions cause a lot of trouble, particularly for those for whom English is not a first language (and often to those for whom it is). For a start, there seem to be no apparent rules, which leads to all kinds of traps, such as *die of* (not *from*), *bored with* (not *of*), *dissent to* (not *from*). Then some verbs will take different prepositions for different meanings: a *taste* for *sardines* is not the same as *a taste of sardines* (and the latter may linger a little longer).

Agree on (a point)	Agree to (a proposal)
Compare with – liken A to B	Compare to – note both resemblance and difference
Correspond to (a thing)	Correspond with (a person)
Differ from (comparisons)	Differ with (someone)
Impatient for (something)	Impatient with (someone)
Part from (a person)	Part with (a thing)

Useful grammatical terms

There are countless (generally impenetrable) books on grammar, so this is a brief guide. But again it should give you more words with which to counter the bluffers, and perhaps help you to understand a bit more of what is going on.

Phrase: A group of words that forms a unit, often without a verb: *the pile of CVs, a constant pressure, a protocol for job appraisal.*

Clause: A group of words with a verb, as in: *The pile of CVs blew away.*

Subordinate clause: A subordinate clause expands on a main clause. It is a group of words with a verb, but clearly not the main part of the sentence: *. . . which was high . . .*

Sentence: A self-contained group of words, with a verb. It starts with a capital letter (*see* below) and ends with a full stop (*see* below): *Everyone ignored the pile of CVs, which was high.*

Subject: The main 'actor' of an active sentence: She *opened the window.* They *closed the door.* It *blew open again.*

Object: The thing that receives the action of the verb. *She opened the* window. *They closed the* door. *It hit my* toe.

Tense: This enables the verb to give us a time frame. There are about 25 tenses, but happily these are divided into three main groups: present – *I am at a meeting*; future – *I will be at a meeting*; past – *I was at a meeting, I had been at a meeting.*

Voice: This refers to whether a verb is in the active or passive (and is often confused with *tense*). The active voice is when the subject does something to the object, as here: *We recommend the cottage pie.* With the passive voice the object becomes the subject, as in: *The cottage pie is recommended by us.* Most people (with the exception of scientists, doctors and bureaucrats/politicians with something to hide) prefer the former: it is shorter, more direct and (here's the rub) much less vague – and therefore harder to wriggle out of.

Subjunctive mood: This is a special form of a verb that indicates something that is possibility rather than fact, or something that is imagined or wished. *If I were a rich woman.* (rather than *If I was a rich woman*). Probably falling into misuse (*see* list 13, below).

Direct and reported speech: Direct speech is within quotation marks (*see* below) and is expected to be an accurate and full account of what was said (or written). Reported speech, while still being accurate, is not necessarily word-for-word or complete. Direct speech: *He said, 'I really must quit this place.'* Reported (indirect) speech: *He said he had to leave.*

Gerund: A verb turned into a noun by adding *-ing*: For example, in *They are waiting, waiting* is a verb. In *I will do the waiting* or *do you mind my waiting while you finish your coffee, waiting* is a gerund.

Simile: Describing something by likening it to something else: *This hospital is like a hotel* or *This office is like a hospital.*

Metaphor: Describing something by calling it something else: *the flagship hospital.*

Syntax: Grammatical structure in sentences, as opposed to parts of speech. The difference between *He was often not on time* and *he was not often on time* is syntactical.

Tautology: Saying the same thing twice, as in *minute detail*. (For more examples *see* page 122.)

Hyperbole: Major exaggeration. *Management accountants are wonderful, the audit was a triumph, we are passionate about double-entry bookkeeping.*

Solecism: Posh word for language error.

TRICKY BIT: WRITING BULLET POINT LISTS

Many people use lists, but not all of them know how to punctuate them properly. This is the way I prefer:

▌ use a colon to start the list (at the end of the lead-in sentence);

▌ do not use a capital letter for the first word of each bullet point

(except for proper nouns) even though Americans and Microsoft like you to do so;
▌ use a series of commas or colons at the end of each line; and
▌ put a full stop at the end of the last point.

The publishers of this book prefer another way, which is to leave the punctuation off the ends of all the lines except the last, which takes a full stop. If the sentence before the bullet list ends in a full stop, or the bulleted lists begins immediately after a heading, they like to start each bullet point with a capital letter and end each bullet point with a full stop.

Punctuation

Punctuation marks may be small, but their influence is great. Take this sentence, for instance: *The managers who came late left the meeting* is not the same as *The managers, who came late, left the meeting*. *The managers, who came late left the meeting* is ambiguous. Punctuation gives the reader important information (instructions, even) on how the words should be read.

Capital letters [C]: Not really a punctuation mark, but vital in telling us when a sentence is beginning. They are also used for proper names. Some people overuse capitals by putting them on any word that they think is important or want to draw attention to.

Full stops [.]: Vital in telling us when a sentence has ended, as in: *This is a simple self-contained sentence.* If an entire sentence is in parentheses, the full stop goes inside the last parenthesis.

Question marks [?]: Used instead of a full stop when a question has been asked: *Agreed?* (as opposed to *Agreed*). *Is the ambulance ready? Why not?*

Exclamation marks (!): The proper use is to signal an exclamation (*Alas! Goodness me! Not likely!*). Often they are used to signal jokes (but if a joke needs signalling, it should probably be left out).

Commas [,]: Sign of a small break or pause in a list: *keys, passport, money and mobile phone.* In UK usage there is no comma before the *and*; in US usage there is: *keys, passport, money, and mobile phone.* This extra comma in a list is called an 'Oxford' or 'serial' comma.

Commas are also used with a conjunction to link two independent clauses (clauses that can both function as sentences on their own): *The departments are on different sites, and communication suffers as a result.* Another use for the comma is to set apart a phrase: *On the appointed day, the patient did not turn up,* or, *The patient, whose time-keeping skills were flawed, failed to turn up.*

Colons [:]: These are used to denote that there is something coming, such as a list or explanation: *We took to the meeting a number of things: handouts, PowerPoint, marker pens, timers, and sandwiches*; or, *The study failed for one reason: too many people had to withdraw.*

Semi colons [;]: One straightforward use is in lists with many words in each item (*see* below). When used between two clauses, it also denotes a pause longer than that of a comma, but shorter than that of a full stop; in other words the writer wants to show that two ideas are closely linked (as in the present sentence). It can be difficult to use, and is not really necessary.

Round brackets/parentheses [()]: Usually used for an aside. *The new consultant (who had only been appointed two weeks previously) decided to defer the meeting.*

Square brackets ([]): Often used to denote references. Also used within inverted commas (*see* below) to show when the original text has been altered: *'He said that [the biologists] had gone away.'*

Dashes [–]: Single dashes are used like a colon, to emphasise drama: *Guess what we found when we got there – a half peeled orange.* Doubles can have the same function as a pair of commas or parentheses: *The greengrocer, who we hoped would come on Tuesday – and preferably even earlier – with the oranges, did not appear in the catering office until Friday.* Many people use hyphens for dashes – note that proper dashes are longer than hyphens.

Bullet points: Also called blobs. These are really a typographical device, not punctuation. When working out the correct punctuation for a bullet pointed list, imagine that the list is really a normal sentence or series of sentences. *See* 'Tricky bit: writing bullet point lists' on page 110.

Inverted commas [' "]: These denote speech or a quotation. Some publications prefer one ('), and others prefer two ("). Look and see what is appropriate.

Hyphens [-]: Used to indicate where two words are particularly related. Hyphens are useful for avoiding confusion: *More-qualified* *doctors* or *more qualified doctors.*

Ellipses [...]: The posh name for three dots. First use is to indicate suspense. *And the winner is . . . John Smith.* Second use is to show that something has been left out: *'I would like to thank many people . . . but the most important is my agent, said John Smith.*

TRICKY BIT: APOSTROPHES

The apostrophe has two main functions. The first one indicates ownership (the possessive). If the owning word ends in *s*, add an apostrophe; if it doesn't end in *s*, add an *'s*: *St James', the manager's office, the patient's complaint, the clinic's waiting room.* Where there is more than one owner the apostrophe comes after the s, as the *managers' meeting, the patients' complaints and the clinics' waiting rooms.*

With a singular noun: add apostrophe, then *'s*. (*a clinic's waiting room, a patient's temperature*). With a plural noun that already ends in *s*: add an apostrophe after the last *s* (*patients' rights, two weeks' wait*).

With a plural noun that doesn't end in *s*: add an apostrophe, then *s* (*the children's ward, women's rights*).

The second function of the apostrophe is indicating if one or more letters have been left out of a word: *hasn't (has not), it's (it is), Middlesboro'* (as a short form of Middlesborough).

The two main errors are: inserting an apostrophe when it is not needed, because the word is a plural, as in *apple's* or *pear's* (this is rather insultingly known as the greengrocer's apostrophe); and getting *it's* and *its* confused: *it's one simple principle* and *its one simple principle.* (The first is a short form of it is; the second is a possessive.)

LIST 5

Words often misspelled

accommodation, not accomodation

admissible, not admissable

argument, not arguement

authoritative, not authoritive

benefited, not benefitted

committee, not commitee

consensus, not concensus

definitely, not definately

diarrhoea, not diarhoea, or dire rear

desperate, not desparate

dissatisfaction, not disatisfaction

ecstasy, not ecstacy or extasy

embarrass, not embarass

fulfilling, not fullfilling

forty, not fourty

grammar, not grammer

harass, not harrass

humorous, not humourous

independent, not independant

indispensable, not indispensible

inoculate, not innoculate

liaise, not liase

maintenance, not maintainance

millennium, not milennium

minuscule, not miniscule

noticeable, not noticable

occurred, not occured

omitted, not omited

ophthalmology, not opthalmology

privilege, not priviledge

profession, not proffession

publicly, not publically

pursue, not persue

restaurateur, not restauranteur

resuscitate, not resusitate

separate, not seperate

straitjacket, not straightjacket

supersede, not supercede

targeted, not targetted

unnecessary, not uneccesary

unparalleled, not unparalelled

veterinary, not vetinerary

withhold, not withold

Perilous pairs

Some words sound the same, but aren't. (If you want to show off, use the word **homophone** to describe them.) The *Guardian's* 'Corrections and Clarifications' column has long been tracking these, and coming up with such gems as *Britain is taking the root pioneered in the US; . . . the original farming, fishing and fouling hamlet*; or *. . . loud-mouthed and chauvinistic boars.*

aural: to do with the ear
born: come into existence
canon: senior clergyman, set of rules
chord: set of musical notes
complement: add to, complete
council: decision-making body
discreet: prudent
enquire: seek information
everyone: all the people
foreword: introductory remarks
formally: according to rules
principal: main (first) person
review: assessment
sight: vision
stationary: still

oral: to do with the mouth
borne: carried
cannon: big gun

cord: string or rope
compliment: praise
counsel: advice, to give advice
discrete: separate
inquire: hold investigation
every one: every person or thing
forward: onward movement
formerly: in the past
principle: rule or guideline
revue: theatrical show
site: place
stationery: writing material

More perilous pairs

These words may not sound the same, but are often confused with each other.

affect: to influence (a verb) **effect:** an outcome (a noun)
appraise: to estimate **apprise:** to inform
biannual: twice a year **biennial:** every two years
contagious: spread by contact **infectious:** spread by air and water
dependant: somebody who is dependent **dependent:** depending on

disinterested: not biased **uninterested:** not interested in
ensure: make sure that **insure:** protect against possible loss
imply: hint **infer:** deduce
impractical: not easy to do **impracticable:** impossible to do
ingenious: clever **ingenuous:** open
journalese: writing style in (some) media **journalism:** collecting and writing news
militate: tell against **mitigate:** appease, make less serious
nauseated: feeling sick **nauseous:** causing sickness
perpetrate: commit **perpetuate:** preserve
prescribe: recommend **proscribe:** forbid
prostate: gland **prostrate:** lying flat
simple: easily understood **simplistic:** excessively simple
tortuous: full of turns **torturous:** painful

Even more perilous pairs (international division)

UK English and US English are, on the whole, similar. But there are some words that, if misused, could get the speaker or writer into some difficulty. This was the case for the US pilot who alarmed his British passengers by saying he was going to land *momentarily*.

	UK English	US English
bill	request for payment	banknote
call	telephone someone	pay a visit
cuffs	turn-up on trousers	turn-up on shirt
dresser	furniture for crockery, etc.	chest of drawers for clothes
homely	pleasant-looking	plain-looking
knock up	waken someone	get someone pregnant
momentarily	for a moment	in a moment
pants	underpants	trousers
pissed	drunk	angry
rubber	eraser	condom
slate	verbally attack	put on list, nominate

Posh words (and their less pompous equivalents)

The words on the right came down from the northern tribes and were used in the meeting houses. Those on the left came up from the Mediterranean, and were used in the counting houses. Other things being equal, use the ones on the right.

accordingly	so
accommodate	hold
additional	more, extra
apparent	clear
approximately	about
ascertain	find out
attempt	try
category	group
commencement	start
deceased	dead
demonstrate	show
discontinue	stop
determine	decide
endeavour	try
exceedingly	very
expenditure	spending
frequently	often
implement	use
location	site, place
peruse	read

purchase	buy
proliferation	spread
remainder	rest
remuneration	pay
subsequently	later
sufficient	enough
terminate	stop
venue	site

Clichés

All clichés were once new and elegant phrases (*see* metaphor, p. 110), but now they are used endlessly. In spoken English, they have their advantages, such as providing an easy and quick way of getting your point across. But when it comes to written English, they should be avoided, because they look tired and unoriginal. It's better to invent your own phrases.

add value
at the end of the day
beggars description
bring up to speed
can of worms
conspicuous by its absence
fall between two stools
given the green light
gold standard
heartfelt thanks
hit the ground running
inextricably linked
in the final analysis
iron out the problem

left up in the air
marked improvement
move the goal posts
paramount importance
sea change
square peg in a round hole
the vast majority
the write stuff
touch base
wealth of information
window of opportunity
win-win situation
without further ado

Redundant words

Many linguists agree that padding is helpful when we are speaking. But when it comes to writing, economy is the key. This means taking many of our favourite spoken phrases and cutting them down to their bare essentials. The words in bold add to the text; the others do not.

adequate enough
appoint to the post of
best ever
collaborate together
consensus of opinion
continue to **remain**
end **result**
entirely **absent**
evidence base
few in number
free **gift**
from **whence**
future **prospect**
gathered together
general **public**
grateful **thanks**
in the course of the **operation**
in conjunction **with**

join together
last of all
major **breakthrough**
may possibly
minute **detail**
needless to say
on a **part time** basis
passing **phase**
past **history**
patently **obvious**
physiotherapist by profession
planning ahead
proposed **project**
regular **monthly meetings**
revert back
serious **danger**
small in size
smile on his face

Lost causes

Language is constantly developing (unless it's a dead one like Latin), so the strictures of grammarians must sometimes make way for what is happening on the streets. Below are some grammatical points that used to be taken seriously; now they have to a greater or lesser extent been overtaken by usage. Pedants will be unhappy, but as Bill Bryson says in his introduction to *The Penguin Dictionary of Troublesome Words*, 'Those who sniff decay in every shift of sense or alteration of usage do the language no service.'

Anticipate: Used to mean look forward to; now means expect.

Decimate: Used to mean kill one in ten (from a Roman custom); now means kill a lot.

First or firstly: Which version to use exercises a fair amount of heat. Most commentators say it doesn't really matter.

Hopefully: To the purists, this means with hope. So *hopefully I will pass my exam* would mean *I will pass my exam with hope* rather than *I hope I will pass my exam*. Usage seems to have moved on, and the second meaning seems to be sticking.

However: Some feel that this should never appear at the start of the sentence. However, it does, quite often.

Over/more than: There are some (including myself) who feel affronted when the word *over* is used with numbers, e.g. *we fly to over 60 countries*. Most authorities now say that this was never really a rule, and that *Over 20 people fell ill* is as acceptable as *More than 20 people fell ill*.

Partial: Strictly speaking, partial means 'biased' (the opposite to impartial), but now it is used to mean in part, e.g. *the bridge was partially submerged*.

Quotation marks and full stops: There is a fiddly rule that editors adhere to, but most others seem ignorant of. Quotation marks should go outside the full stop if the quoted material is a complete sentence (with initial capital letter). He said, *'The negotiations were a waste of time.'* but *He said the negotiations were 'a waste of time'*. To make things more confusing, the Americans always put the quote marks after the full stop.

Sex: There are some who insist that **gender** is a term of grammar, and therefore we should talk about male and female sex, rather than gender. This battle seems to have been lost.

Shall and will: Another area where pedants like to roam. Again, take comfort from the wise words of Bill Bryson: 'To try and formulate rules here would be a dangerous and perhaps impossible exercise.'

Split infinitive: You split an infinitive when you put an adverb between the two parts of a verb, as in *to* boldly *go*. Generations of English speakers have been brought up to believe that this is forbidden. All commentators agree that it is not, nor should it be. As Kingsley Amis wrote, it is 'the best known of the imaginary rules that petty linguistic tyrants seek to lay on the English language'.

Racist and sexist words you can't print

The wonderful world of style

Here is a fairly idiosyncratic list of points that have exercised me – and course participants – over the years.

Amongst, whilst: Prefer *among* and *while*. Kingsley Amis says that they are 'not to be used unless a fussy old-fashioned air should for some reason be aimed at'.

Avoid (as in *avoid alcohol*)**:** What does it mean?

Bi- (as in montly, weekly, annual)**:** What does this mean: twice a week or every two weeks? Best to be clear: *twice a week, every two weeks,* etc.

Centre around: A contradiction if you think about it; use *centre on*.

Christian names: Inappropriate in today's multicultural society; prefer *first name*.

Common sense: Useful when writing, so that you can avoid terms such as *whole half chicken*.

Compliance: A horribly value-laden word to describe whether people have taken their medicine. Why not, *take their medicine?*

Comprise: Does not need *of*. A list *consists of* several items, but it *comprises* several items.

Data: Scientists insist it is plural, with datum being the singular, though this seems to have become a bit of an affectation. Grammarians say it can be treated as a collective noun, and thereby take the singular (*data is . . .*). Agenda, however, is always singular.

Decorated municipal gothic: Term coined by Dr Michael O'Donnell to describe what happens when people abandon simple writing. Allegedly inspired by notice: *This dustcart is being utilised for highway cleansing purposes.*

Female, Male: Women and men sometimes do as well, if not better.

First person *(I did this, we did that)***:** There was a time when it was frowned upon, especially in science. But the tide is turning, and many people (editors particularly) say that if you did it, you should say so and not hide behind a passive (*It was done*).

Full stops and abbreviations: The current trend is not to use these together. Thus we have *the BBC, Mr, Prof.*

GPs: This is the plural of GP. GP's (and GPs') is the possessive. Thus *The GPs complained about their contract* but *The GPs' contract was not signed because of a single GP's complaint.*

Home in on: Not *hone in on.*

Lay people: A bit snooty (after all, you are a lay person when you are reading this book). Prefer *public.*

Livid: Originally meant leaden or grey coloured. Now seems to mean red with anger.

Misplaced modifier: A phrase that has wandered off to the wrong part of the sentence, thereby changing the meaning: *the patient was found by the nurse with a bedpan between his legs.*

Mixed metaphor: Can get you into trouble, as in *he was left to paddle his own canoe up a one-way street* or *he sank the project by moving the goal posts.*

Monologophobia: The fear of using the same word twice. Can lead to heroic efforts to avoid, which become even more confusing. *The study showed . . . The investigation demonstrated . . . The researches also revealed . . .* Why not: *The researches showed three things . . .?*

Nice: Weedy and vague. Find a more precise word.

Noun salads: As in: *The Red Book residual list size arithmetic rules.* Deconstruct.

Nouning: Turning good verbs into nouns: *we discussed the implementation of the report* is not as effective as: *We discussed implementing the report* (which probably accounts for its popularity in bureaucratic circles).

Patronising: Some people worry that if they use short words and simple sentences they will come across as patronising. That is not a concern shared by the tabloid newspapers. What is patronising, however, is using phrases such as: *as we doctors/nurses/physios call it*, and *lay people.*

Pompous initial capitals: The habit of awarding capital letters to oneself and one's organisation. The *Health Worker, Hospital Authorities* and *Unit*. This is also patronising (*see* above).

Sexist language: Many authorities now say that it is all right to use the plural *they/them* as a singlar pronoun, instead of *he/him* or *she/her*. For example: *If someone comes in, sit them down.*

Spacing after a full stop: In the days of typewriters (and secretarial academies) it was considered essential to have two spaces after each full stop. Now, with automatic spacing on computers, one is enough.

That, which: *That* is for essential information; *which* is for extra information (and is surrounded with commas): *The file that is thick was taken to the meeting* and *The file, which is thick, was taken to the meeting.* In the first version the thick file was specially selected; in the second it happened to be thick.

Try: Takes *to* and not *and*. I will *try to go*, not *try and go*.

Verbing: The habit of turning a good noun into a verb: pencil into pencilled, for instance. But it can get out of hand, giving us a word like *overshoeshopped* and a phrase like *waked and buried.*

Very: Overdone. Use occasionally. (And do not use *exceedingly* as a substitute.)

Ten sensible principles (and the results of ignoring them)

1 **Once you have written something, read it back to see what you have really said . . .**
   'The second sister underwent hysterectomy at age 40, while still cycling.' – *draft of scientific paper*
   'The patient complained about nausea, pain and sudden death.' – *reported by course participant*
   'Three years have passed since your angioplasty. So it is time for your annual check-up.' – *letter to the politician Roy Hattersley, reported in the* GUARDIAN
   'In the event of a terminal evacuation . . .' – *notice in lavatory at Gatwick Airport*

2 **. . . and whether you really want to say it**
   'If door is closed please wait outside.' – *notice at hospital*
   'Towels are for the use of the Chief Executive only. All others please use paper towels.' – *personal communication*
   'Take two days running then skip a day.' – *prescription advice*

3 **Watch the punctuation**
   'Anyone who is concerned about the speech and language, or swallowing of a family member, or themselves, is welcome to attend an open day.' – *from medical school press release*
   'New drug overcomes GP's main problem in managing unstable bladder.' – *newsletter*

4 **Watch the word order**

'[He] wants all primary care trust public health directors to contact local MPs to spell out the benefits of a total ban on the population's health.' – *Health Service Journal*

'He got into a row with a 35-year-old man who lived nearby over dog faeces.' – *Leatherhead Advertiser*

5 **Don't trust the spell-check**

'Symptoms were relived in 31 [patients].' – *BMJ*

'They are very tight lipped, but believe it will be a major leaver in prompting government action.' – *Health Services Journal*

'I am confident that these changes will provide many exiting opportunities for staff.' – *management handout.*

'I do not demure from any of these messages.' – *Training Journal*

'His health worsened considerably during the final months of his life and the Fund did all it could to elevate his suffering.' – *draft article for charity newsletter*

6 **Avoid science speak**

'There were no conversions during surgery.' – *course participant*

'Malnutrition adversely affects survival among young adults.' – *course participant*

'You are being invited to take part in a non-invasive and ionising radiation free arteriovenous fistulae surveillance study.' – *contributed anonymously*

7 **Be sparing with initials**

NHS R&D NCCHTA

'HSJ understands that the NHSU's renewed efforts to influence SHA MPET funding decisions led to increased tensions across the DoH and SHA "top team".' – *HSJ*

8 **Use real English wherever possible**

'The editors reserve the right to make literary corrections. Please couch terminology so that it will be understood by an international readership.' – *JOURNAL OF PUBLIC HEALTH MEDICINE*

9 **Ask yourself whether you are happy that only two people are likely to understand**

'This study shows that it is possible for medical practitioners to problematise the Cartesianism of biomedicine and its effects on both patients and doctors, and to conceptualise the integrative framework encapsulated in the notion of embodiment as lived medicine.' – *Medical Humanities abstract*

'The introduction of clinical governance will require every NHS provider to embrace the need for robust quality improvement processes in their organisation. There is also a determination to drive down management and support costs by abolishing the internal market and encouraging organisations to share support functions.' – *NHS document*

'The self taught package seemed to be more effective (and thus more cost effective for the journal) than the face to face training, although for the review quality instrument this result is only of borderline significance if non-responders are on average editorially significant worse than responders.' – BMJ *(two editors as authors)*

'Supportive counselling is sometimes described and explained in theoretical terms as Rogerian person-centred therapy. Rooted in a non-mechanistic philosophy, person-centred therapy is non manualised and experiential, and core conditions of empathy, acceptance and genuineness are utilised by the therapist within the therapeutic relationship to facilitate the client toward self awareness and self determination.' – *donated copy*

10 Only make it obscure if you really want to

'We are therefore administratively inactivating the application.' (In other words, 'no'.) – *US grant-giving organisation*

'At the heart of the action plan is the recognition that support for the community self-help and grass roots activity is vital if we are to enable communities to contribute to solutions which they are expertly placed to visualise and undertake.' – *source unknown*

'On the balance of probability, one cannot say with 100 per cent certainty that I did not say anything which I would not have said when not under the influence.' – *doctor conducting his own defence at the GMC*

Five to try on your own

Here are some badly written sentences for you to rewrite. Alternatives are given below. These are suggestions only; you may well come up with better solutions.

1 'In order to foster collegiate understanding of individual development proposals, it is suggested that a more detailed consideration is undertaken by our group of individual development proposals.' – *from NHS estates office*

2 'Student performance in the end of year examinations was significantly enhanced in the year of the intervention.' – *Medical Education*

3 'At this early stage in curriculum reform, however, it was understandable that tutor availability was the rate-limiting step and that tutor recruitment prioritised expertise in facilitation.' – *Medical Education*

4 'Female pharmacists' labour participation rates in the workforce are lower than their male counterparts. In particular, female pharmacists, in common with other female workers, are much more likely to work part-time than their male counterparts.' – *submission to pharmaceutical journal*

5 'The whole purpose of reaching agreement in respect of maintaining disagreements that occur within an internal framework has been known for many years. We would therefore ask you on this occasion as we have asked you in the past to continue to use the further stages in the internal procedure if you so desire in order

that no accusations can be levelled at either side for failing to abide by agreements.' – *BMA document*

SOME SUGGESTED ALTERNATIVES

1 We should discuss the plans again.
2 Students did considerably better that year.
3 The problem at this early stage was not having enough tutors, so teaching them facilitation skills became a priority.
4 Women pharmacists work fewer hours than men pharmacists and are more likely to work part-time.
5 Please follow the internal grievance procedure.

Quotes to drop

PROCESS

- 'Revising is part of writing. Few writers are so expert that they can produce what they are after on the first try.' – *EB White*
- 'Don't get it right, get it written.' – *James Thurber*
- 'Keep it simple. Be clear. Think of your reader, not yourself. Cheer up.' – *Roger Angell*
- 'The only way to write is well and how you do it is your own damn business.' – *AJ Liebling*
- 'What is written without effort is in general read without pleasure.' – *Samuel Johnson*
- 'What can be said at all can be said clearly.' – *Ludwig Wittgenstein*
- 'Get up very early and get going at once; in fact work first and wash afterwards.' – *WH Auden*
- 'For any writer, but for the beginning writer in particular, it's wise to eliminate every possible distraction.' – *Stephen King*
- 'Writing is hard, even for authors who do it all the time.' – *Roger Angell*
- 'When you say something, make sure you have said it. The chances of your having said it are only fair.' – *EB White*

STYLE

- 'Have something to say and say it as clearly as you can. That is the only secret of style.' – *Mathew Arnold*
- Style is 'essentially good manners'. – *Arthur Quiller-Couch*
- 'The full stop is a great help to sanity.' – *Harold Evans*
- 'Read over your compositions, and when you meet a passage that you think is particularly fine, strike it out.' – *Samuel Johnson*
- 'Short words are best, and the old words when short are best of all.' – *Winston Churchill*
- 'Language does not always have to wear a tie and lace-up shoes.' – *Stephen King*
- 'Abstract words should be chased out in favour of specific, concrete words. Sentences should be full of bricks, beds, houses, cars, cows, men and women. Details should drive out generality. And everything should be related to human beings.' – *Harold Evans*
- 'The tragedy of scientific writing is that whole generations of young people who started writing "The cat sat on the mat" and "Mummy is eating an orange" have been forced to write "The mat is sat on by the cat" and "The orange is being eaten by Mummy" because it is more scientific.' – *Richard Smith*
- 'Proper words in proper places make the true definition of style.' – *Jonathan Swift*

GEORGE ORWELL'S MUCH-QUOTED RULES ON STYLE

1 Never use a metaphor, simile or other figure of speech which you are used to seeing in print.
2 Never use a long word where a short one will do.
3 If it is possible to cut a word out, always cut it out.
4 Never use the passive where you can use the active.
5 Never use a foreign phrase, a scientific word or a jargon word if you can think of an everyday British equivalent.
6 Break any of these rules sooner than say anything outright barbaric.

Politics and the English Language, 1946.

LAST WORD

▮ 'I hate writing. Having written is great' – *Tim Albert*

Index

abbreviations and initials 130
adjectives 107
adverbs 107
Angell, Roger 134
apostrophes 114
Arial typeface 91, 95–6
Arnold, Mathew 135
Auden, WH 134
audiences
    identifying 24–6
    importance of 14–15
    multiple readerships 17, 81–2
    targeted writing models 9,
      14–19

balanced feedback structures
  58–60
book chapters, suggested structures
  43–4
brackets 113
Bryson, Bill 123–4
bullet points 91, 94, 110–11, 113

capital letters 64, 91, 97, 112
checking facts 61–2
Churchill, Winston 135
clauses 109

clichés 121
colleagues and peers *see* feedback
colons 113
commas 112–13
conjunctions 108
creative 'flow' 49–50

dashes 113
deadlines 26, 80
design and layout 91–102
direct speech 110
displacement activities
    over editing 85–6
    over researching 9

editing practices 85–6
    see also rewriting
effective writing
    defined 13–14, 19–20
    models 14–19
    outcome benefits 15–17
    and problem feedback 19
ellipses 114
emails, suggested structures
  41–2
Evans, Harold 135
exclamation marks 112